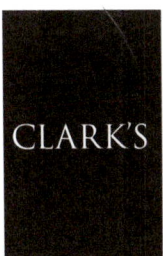

CLARK'S

ESSENTIAL GUIDE TO

PRELIMINARY CLINICAL EVALUATION OF MUSCULOSKELETAL X-RAYS

This easy-to-understand guide in the highly respected Clark's stable of diagnostic imaging texts is an invaluable tool for student and qualified radiographers, providing practical advice and instruction on how to formulate a comment following image evaluation of musculoskeletal X-rays. Covering both trauma and pathology of the musculoskeletal system, the reader can find essential information quickly, with content including key points and take-home messages throughout.

Clark's Essential Guide to Preliminary Clinical Evaluation of Musculoskeletal X-rays takes the systematic approach adopted within books in the Clark's family and is designed to be clear and consistent. Accessible text and high-quality illustration ensure that this book will both educate those practitioners learning to evaluate images and support those doing it routinely in clinical practice. Additionally, the book provides invaluable guidance to those departments that have not yet progressed to commenting but are looking to introduce this by outlining a development plan for staff and suggesting content for any formal documentation that is required.

Clark's Companion Essential Guides

Series Editor
A. Stewart Whitley

https://www.routledge.com/Clarks-Companion-Essential-Guides/book-series/CRCCLACOMESS

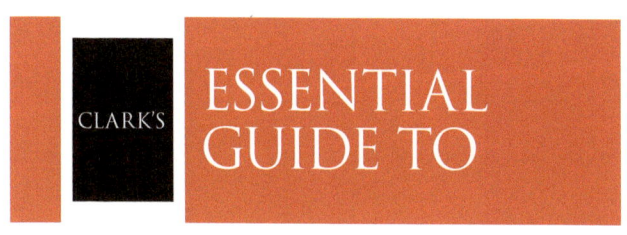

PRELIMINARY CLINICAL EVALUATION OF MUSCULOSKELETAL X-RAYS

Amanda Martin
Radiography Consultant and Lecturer, University of Cumbria, UK

Illustrated by Ruth Eaves
Medical Artist, Royal Bolton Hospital, Bolton NHS Foundation Trust, UK

Series Editor for *Clark's Companion Essential Guides*
A. Stewart Whitley
Radiology Advisor, UK Radiology Advisory Services, Preston, Lancashire, UK, and Former Director of Professional Practice, International Society of Radiographers and Radiological Technologists (ISRRT)

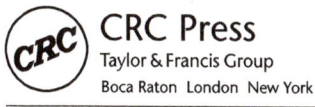

CRC Press is an imprint of the
Taylor & Francis Group, an **informa** business

Designed cover images: Author's own.

First edition published 2025
by CRC Press
2385 NW Executive Center Drive, Suite 320, Boca Raton, FL 33431

and by CRC Press
4 Park Square, Milton Park, Abingdon, Oxon OX14 4RN

CRC Press is an imprint of Taylor & Francis Group, LLC

This book contains information obtained from authentic and highly regarded sources. While all reasonable efforts have been made to publish reliable data and information, neither the author[s] nor the publisher can accept any legal responsibility or liability for any errors or omissions that may be made. The publishers wish to make clear that any views or opinions expressed in this book by individual editors, authors or contributors are personal to them and do not necessarily reflect the views/opinions of the publishers. The information or guidance contained in this book is intended for use by medical, scientific or health-care professionals and is provided strictly as a supplement to the medical or other professional's own judgement, their knowledge of the patient's medical history, relevant manufacturer's instructions and the appropriate best practice guidelines. Because of the rapid advances in medical science, any information or advice on dosages, procedures or diagnoses should be independently verified. The reader is strongly urged to consult the relevant national drug formulary and the drug companies' and device or material manufacturers' printed instructions, and their websites, before administering or utilizing any of the drugs, devices or materials mentioned in this book. This book does not indicate whether a particular treatment is appropriate or suitable for a particular individual. Ultimately it is the sole responsibility of the medical professional to make his or her own professional judgements, so as to advise and treat patients appropriately. The authors and publishers have also attempted to trace the copyright holders of all material reproduced in this publication and apologize to copyright holders if permission to publish in this form has not been obtained. If any copyright material has not been acknowledged please write and let us know so we may rectify in any future reprint.

ISBN: 9781032979465 (hbk)
ISBN: 9781032832920 (pbk)
ISBN: 9781003596264 (ebk)

DOI: 10.1201/9781003596264

Typeset in Linotype Berling LT Std
by Evolution Design & Digital Ltd (Kent)

For Product Safety Concerns and Information please contact our EU representative:
GPSR@taylorandfrancis.com

Taylor & Francis Verlag GmbH, Kaufingerstraße 24, 80331 München, Germany

CONTENTS

Contents

FOREWORD

It has been a delight to witness the development and publication of *Clark's Essential Guide to Preliminary Clinical Evaluation of Musculoskeletal X-rays*.

This latest addition to the *Clark's* series of pocket and desktop books is a testament to the skills, knowledge and dedication of the author, who has at heart a passion to share her knowledge and experience with radiographers engaged in this area of expertise.

Radiographers writing their preliminary clinical evaluation of images to support onward patient management has been a vision of the College of Radiographers since 2013, as outlined in its policy and reinforced in 2024 in the document *Radiographer Preliminary Clinical Evaluation*. This book will provide excellent background knowledge both to preliminary clinical evaluation, across a range of musculoskeletal situations, and to the task of commenting on images, demonstrating how this can be accomplished in a thoughtful and organised way.

Undertaking preliminary clinical evaluation of musculoskeletal X-ray images and composing comments are important aspects of the radiographer's role in the modern generation of the radiography workforce. Not only are these vital aspects of patient care, but they reflect radiographers' understanding of the content of the diagnostic images that they produce. Communicating details of fractures and other pathologies spotted in the images that they produce provides the referring clinician with a wealth of information before a formal report is issued.

Miss K.C. Clark, I am sure, would welcome this important addition to the *Clark's Companion Essential Guides*. I am confident that all involved in the task of evaluating and commenting on musculoskeletal images will benefit greatly from this publication.

A. Stewart Whitley
Series Editor
Former ISRRT Director of Professional Practice &
Radiology Advisor
UK Radiology Advisory Services
Preston, Lancashire, UK

PREFACE

In 2013, the Society and College of Radiographers indicated an expectation that all radiographers would provide preliminary comments on the images that they produce. Undergraduate programmes incorporated the required education for students to be able to fulfil this requirement upon qualification. However, a document published by the Society and College of Radiographers in 2024[1] identified that the introduction of this practice has been sporadic. While it stated that a formal report is the gold standard, it also identified that there are many situations in which there is a delay between the immediate treatment needs of the patient and the issuing of a formal report, making the radiographer's comment a safety net for the referrer.

Commenting on images is a progression from what was traditionally called 'red dotting'. To 'red dot' an image meant that an abnormality had been identified, but specific descriptors were not necessary in documenting what that abnormality was. Texts are available to assist in red dotting or in formal image interpretation, that is, to apply meaning to the abnormality that has been identified and produce a definitive report. The aim of this book is to support radiology departments to introduce a commenting service by outlining the governance associated with it and suggesting content for any formal documentation. In addition, there is evidence that practitioners are not confident in providing comments, with Harcus et al. (2024)[2] identifying that there is a need for training in structuring and writing comments. The book will guide practitioners through the evaluation of the images to the production of comments.

It is difficult in a text such as this to include subtle findings, as image reproduction removes some of the resolution that is available on viewing monitors, imaging tools are not available for manipulation and the images are only small. Where possible, images have been used that easily demonstrate the abnormality being discussed.

Section 1 introduces the basics of a systematic evaluation of images and guide the reader through the structuring of a comment using a template-based approach to develop confidence. It will also explain bone development and decline in bone health, as both have an impact on image appearances. This knowledge will be applied to the paediatric and adult appendicular and axial skeleton in Sections 2, 3 and 4. Given that one of the principles of image evaluation is that the whole image must be reviewed, it is recognised that there is a responsibility for radiographers to identify abnormalities in the chest and abdomen if these are seen on musculoskeletal images. Common pathologies associated with the chest and abdomen are included in the relevant chapters. It may be the case that the pathology identified in the chest or abdomen has greater clinical significance than any seen in the area under investigation, so it is essential that radiographers know when to escalate any abnormal findings and when it is acceptable not to escalate these findings.

Radiographers are in the unique position of being the first person to see a patient's images, and they should have the ability to identify signs of abuse on them so that the appropriate safeguarding processes can be followed. Section 5 presents the radiological signs of abuse in both children and older people. Section 6 presents the most common pathological appearances associated with arthritis, infection and bone lesions, recognising that this book is aimed not at the interpretation of radiological findings in order to reach a diagnosis but at the evaluation of the image for the purpose of escalation of any urgent findings.

Section 7 includes a number of practice cases, each having a small section for the reader to make notes to support evaluation and develop a comment. A detailed approach to evaluation is then presented for each case so that readers can explore their own thought processes, measured against those of an experienced reporting practitioner.

Amanda Martin

References

1. Society and College of Radiographers. *Radiographer Preliminary Clinical Evaluation*. London: Society and College of Radiographers, 2024.
2. Harcus, J., Stevens, B., Pabtic, V. and Hewis, J. Preliminary clinical evaluation: where are we? An international scoping review. *Radiography* 2024;**30**(5):1474–1482.

ACKNOWLEDGEMENTS

I am indebted to many people for their support throughout my extensive career in radiography, from those who patiently trained me as a student to those who believed in me when I embarked on a pilot programme for radiographer reporting in 1995. Throughout my career, projectional radiography, and in particular musculoskeletal imaging, has been my passion, and I have been fortunate enough to be supported by some of the best in the profession. Dr Nigel Thomas, Consultant Radiologist, was an advocate for radiographer reporting right from the start and, while I will never reach the dizzying heights of his level of knowledge, I feel privileged that he was able to share at least some of his knowledge with me in my early reporting days. Later in my career, Dr Rakesh Mehan, Consultant Radiologist, has been an amazing mentor; I am sure that there is nothing that he does not know about musculoskeletal imaging.

Jeremy Weldon, Consultant Radiographer, started the journey of this book with me many years ago. When circumstances changed and Jeremy withdrew from the writing, he allowed me to continue to use some of his work on chest and facial bone imaging and for that I am extremely grateful. Samantha Mahgoub and Mohammed Bhana, Reporting Radiographers, have helped me in the completion of this book, sense checking what I was writing when I was at risk of becoming word blind. Teaching images have been contributed by several people.

I must thank A. Stewart Whitley, Series Editor, for putting his trust in my ability to produce a book that may be useful to the profession going forwards. His tenacious approach to the education of our future radiographers goes unmatched.

I am privileged to have one of the country's best Medical Artists, Ruth Eaves, as a personal friend. Her award-winning artwork has brought my book to life and it has been an absolute pleasure working on this book together.

Acknowledgements

My most heartfelt thanks go to my family: to my son, my proudest achievement by far, and my husband, who have both never questioned my impulsiveness when I take on a challenge or doubted my ability to complete it, and have supported me by giving me the time and space, the IT support, the hot drinks and the chocolate when times have been tough; to my sister, who has kept me grounded by sharing her craziness with me; and, finally, to my parents, who instilled in me the belief that I can achieve anything I set out to achieve, who taught me to be the best that I can be and who gave me the confidence to succeed.

ABBREVIATIONS

ACJ	acromioclavicular joint
AIIS	anterior inferior iliac spine
AP	anteroposterior
ASIS	anterior superior iliac spine
CDH	congenital dislocation of the hip
CMCJ	carpometacarpal joint
CRITOE	capitellum, radial head, internal epicondyle, trochlea, olecranon, external epicondyle
CT	computed tomography
DDH	developmental dysplasia of the hip
DHS	dynamic hip screw
DIPJ	distal interphalangeal joint
DISH	diffuse idiopathic skeletal hyperostosis
DP	dorsi-palmar/dorsi-plantar
DRUJ	distal radio-ulna joint
ED	Emergency Department
FOOSH	fall onto the outstretched hand
GHJ	glenohumeral joint
MC	metacarpal
MSK	musculoskeletal
MT	metatarsal
OA	osteoarthritis
OPG	orthopantomogram
PIPJ	proximal interphalangeal joint
RA	rheumatoid arthritis
SCIWORA	spinal cord injury without radiographic abnormality
SCJ	sternoclavicular joint
SH	Salter–Harris
SUFE	slipped upper (or proximal) femoral epiphysis
TMJ	temporomandibular joint
TMTJ	tarsometatarsal joint

SECTION 1
INTRODUCTION

1. INTRODUCTION TO COMMENTING

On 8 November 1895, Wilhelm Conrad Röntgen discovered a new kind of radiation that could penetrate the body and produce an image of the skeleton. As the use of ionising radiation for medical purposes evolved, the distinction between radiographer and radiologist developed,[1] and for the greatest part of the subsequent years there was much debate about which profession should interpret these images and provide a report. However, studies in the 1970s concluded that, with adequate training and appropriate delegation, radiographers could report on selected images to the same level as radiologists.[2-4] Around this time, a scheme was gaining popularity in which a **red dot** was applied to an image if the radiographer identified an abnormality.[5] This led to a reduction in missed abnormalities in the Emergency Department (ED), but this method was non-specific, as it did not indicate the location of the abnormality. Although there was support from the professional bodies for this process, it did not extend to radiographers issuing formal reports.

As radiologist numbers were decreasing, workforce pressures were increasing due to new technologies, such as computed tomography (CT), which required more time for image interpretation. In addition, the backlog of 'plain film' reporting was increasing. The Audit Commission suggested reporting by radiographers as a solution to this crisis.[6] Despite this being rejected by the professional and regulatory bodies,[7,8] some radiologists developed programmes to determine if focused training on image interpretation would enable radiographers to develop competencies in reporting. These were successful, and formal **independent reporting** by radiographers commenced in the 1990s. As this became established, the College of Radiographers indicated that there should be progression from applying red dots to offering a **preliminary clinical evaluation**, also known as a **comment**, on images[9,10] and undergraduate education programmes changed to reflect this.

Commenting by radiographers is in its infancy and there is reluctance to engage with it by some. However, if good governance is followed, there is no reason why it cannot become an established part of day-to-day practice.

GOOD GOVERNANCE

Commenting is a natural development from the 'red dot' scheme and involves documenting the findings of an **evaluation** of the images, carried out for the purposes of identifying an abnormality or indicating that no abnormality has been seen. Making that move from 'red dotting' to commenting can be challenging for those who may be concerned about the legality of providing a comment. While the comment constitutes a report in the pedantic sense, it is not a formal, legally binding report, and the referrer is still responsible for fully evaluating the images in line with national legislation.[11] A **formal report** is issued only once the findings of the evaluation have been **interpreted (Table 1.1)**. A statement alongside the comment indicating that a formal report will follow is recommended.

If the lack of commenting is due to low confidence, consider auditing red dot accuracy and delivering training where needed. In addition, reporting radiographers could provide individualised feedback on comments provided by radiographers.

Providing a comment on normal images, such as 'no apparent abnormality' or 'no abnormality detected', requires some consideration, as providing referrers with assistance in the identification of normal appearances is just as important as that for abnormal appearances. However, there can be some hesitation in indicating normality because of the possible consequences of getting this wrong. If this is the case, consider asking a reporting radiographer to **audit** red dot accuracy and provide training where needed.

Good governance associated with commenting includes as a minimum:

- identifying that the image for commenting is from an **approved referral source**; for example, comments may be limited to referrals from the ED or extended to other sources;

Table 1.1 Summary of the key concepts of evaluating, commenting and reporting.

Process	Definition	Example
Evaluating	Assessing an image to identify an abnormality	A lucent area is seen in the distal tibia.
Red dotting	Application of an electronic red dot to the image, indicating that an abnormality is present	A red dot is applied, indicating that a lucent area has been seen.
Commenting	Provision of a comment about the abnormality seen	A comment is made stating that a lucent area has been seen in the distal tibia.
Interpretation	Assigning meaning to the results of the evaluation by interpreting the findings and reaching a diagnosis	The appearances associated with the lucent area are interpreted and a diagnosis is made of a benign non-ossifying fibroma.
Reporting	Formally documenting the results of the interpretation to facilitate patient management	A formal report is issued stating that a benign non-ossifying fibroma is present in the distal tibia.

- ensuring that the comment is made within the agreed **scope of practice**; this may vary between different settings but must include as a minimum:

  - the age range of patients whose images may be commented on;
  - the anatomical areas to be included in the commenting system;
  - the types of abnormalities that are appropriate for commenting, such as acute and healing fractures, subluxations, dislocations, foreign body retention, effusion or lipohaemarthrosis, chest infection, pneumothorax or perforation;

- exclusion criteria, such as comments not being made on arthritis in an older patient, benign bone lesions or known conditions such as lung fibrosis.

- reviewing previous images, when possible, to determine if a finding is acute or chronic;
- conducting self-audits to identify areas that may need improvement, and accessing the appropriate training to improve commenting practices;
- accessing a reporting practitioner to expedite an urgent formal report for a clinically significant finding or to speak directly with the referrer if a finding needs immediate clinical intervention; local protocols must be followed but some examples of clinically urgent findings are:

  - a tension pneumothorax in an acutely unwell patient in the ED;
  - a suspicious lung lesion on the chest X-ray of a general practitioner (GP)'s patient that may require urgent CT imaging;
  - an incorrectly positioned endotracheal, nasogastric or nasojejunal tube;
  - infective signs such as osteomyelitis;
  - aggressive lesions that have not previously been documented or have progressed since previous imaging.

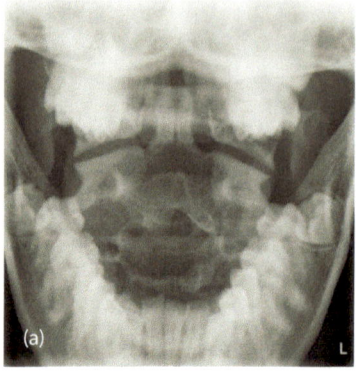 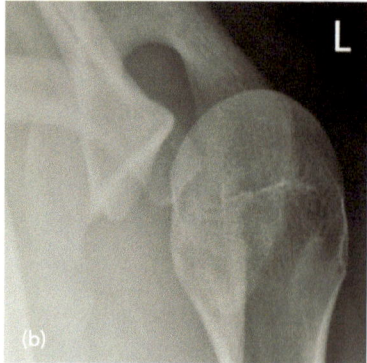

Figure 1.1 (a) A Mach effect lucency caused by the incisors on the odontoid peg image. (b) Posterior dislocation on an axial shoulder image – the humeral head has moved towards the acromion process.

BASICS OF EVALUATION

Before being able to identify an abnormality, there must be good knowledge of normal three-dimensional paediatric and adult anatomy and how this presents on a two-dimensional image. This will allow correct interpretation of signs such as overlapping structures, referred to as a Mach effect (**Figure 1.1a**), and enable correct identification of the direction of a dislocated joint, such as the shoulder (**Figure 1.1b**).

In addition, an understanding of soft tissue anatomy is important.

- It will help identify the subtle non-bony signs of **radiologically occult fractures**, where a fracture is not visible on the image. This may be an effusion or a lipohaemarthrosis, for example.
- Atraumatic pain may be associated with tendon calcification, and knowledge of tendon location will support such a diagnosis.
- An understanding of chest and abdomen anatomy will help in the appreciation of lung and abdominal pathologies, which may be visualised on musculoskeletal (MSK) images. It is useful to have some knowledge of evaluation of these areas. This will be discussed in more detail in the relevant chapters.

This chapter will focus on the general systematic method for evaluating all MSK images, with further details related to individual body parts discussed in subsequent chapters. When looking at images, appropriate viewing conditions are needed. Glare from lights on monitors can be distracting, as can evaluating images while chatting with colleagues. In daily practice, the images are likely to be evaluated in the X-ray room, and this may make controlling the environment difficult. Where possible, identify a separate location that is quiet and has subdued lighting.

Not everybody will evaluate the bones and joints in the same order, but maintaining consistency in the way that you do this will result in an improvement in accuracy and speed of evaluation. A systematic method ensures that every aspect of the image is scrutinised for an abnormality. The MSK system is evaluated using the **ABCs method**,[12] and this is applied regardless of which part of the skeleton is being evaluated. The original method has been adapted slightly to reflect the thought process that takes place when looking at images:

- A adequacy;
- B bones;
- C cartilaginous areas, including growth plates and joint spaces;
- S soft tissues, including those within the lungs and abdomen;
- S satisfaction of search.

Assessment of Adequacy

Checking the adequacy of images is the first step of evaluation, as errors can be made if images are inadequate. Poor patient preparation, technique, choice of projections and exposure factors are the main causes of inadequate images.

- **Patient preparation** is essential, and this includes the removal of all artefacts from the region of interest. Hair, jewellery, clothing and echocardiogram electrodes can all have an impact on diagnosis by obscuring a pathology or causing distortion within the soft tissues (**Figure 1.2**). In addition, a lack of inspiration can hide a lesion on a chest image, so good instruction on breathing should be given before exposure (**Figure 1.3**).

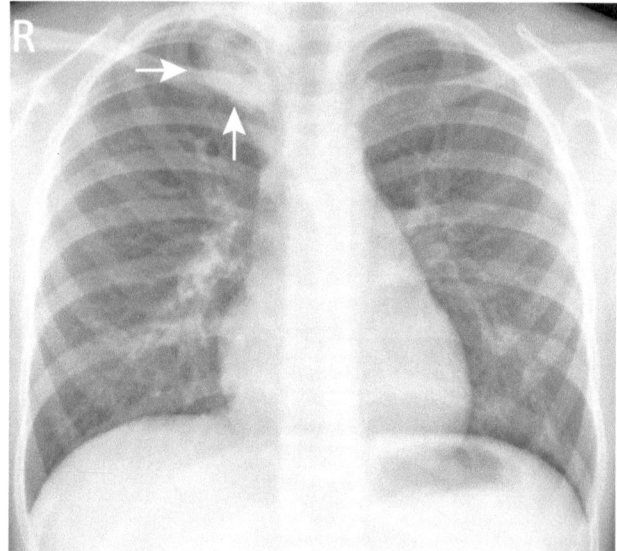

Figure 1.2 Chest image demonstrating hair artefact in the right apex looking like a lung lesion.

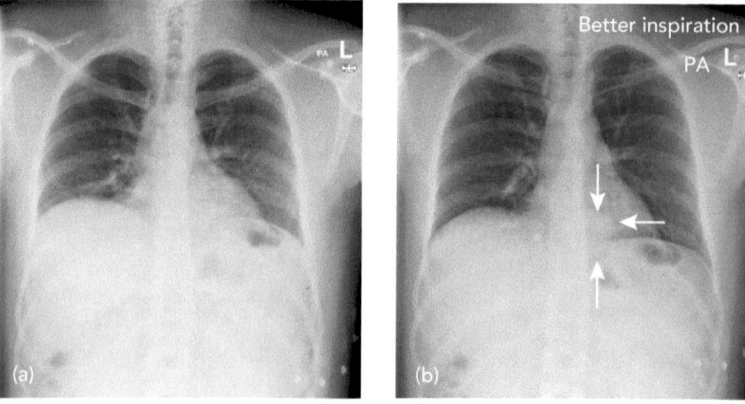

Figure 1.3 Chest images demonstrating (a) a lack of inspiration and (b) a lesion behind the heart when exposure is taken on improved inspiration.

■ **Exposure factors** may have an impact on your ability to see an abnormality. Overexposure may result in obliteration of soft tissues (**Figure 1.4a**), while underexposure will not demonstrate adequate bony detail (**Figure 1.4b**). It is better to set the correct exposure factors than to rely on image manipulation tools during post-processing.

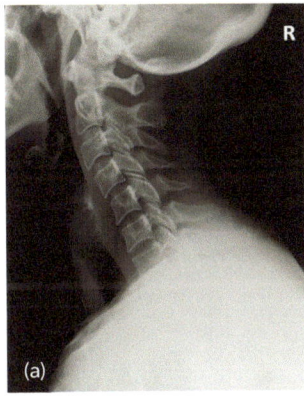 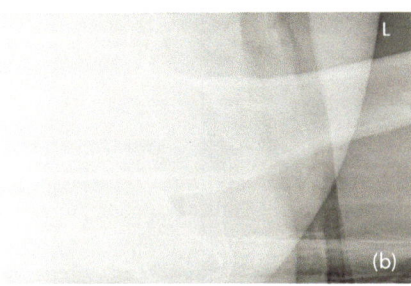

Figure 1.4 (a) Lateral cervical spine image demonstrating the effect of overexposure on soft tissue detail. (b) Lateral hip image demonstrating poor bony detail due to underexposure.

■ **Projections and techniques** have been developed and standardised worldwide to best demonstrate anatomical structures, and using these provides the greatest chance of identifying an abnormality. The clinical indication must direct the choice of projections; for example, hand projections obtained for a thumb injury will not clearly demonstrate trauma to the thumb or first metacarpal. It is crucial to focus on technical accuracy in all situations, including when carrying out challenging examinations (**Figure 1.5**). Abnormalities will be missed if the correct projections are not obtained and/or they are not technically correct (**Figure 1.6**).

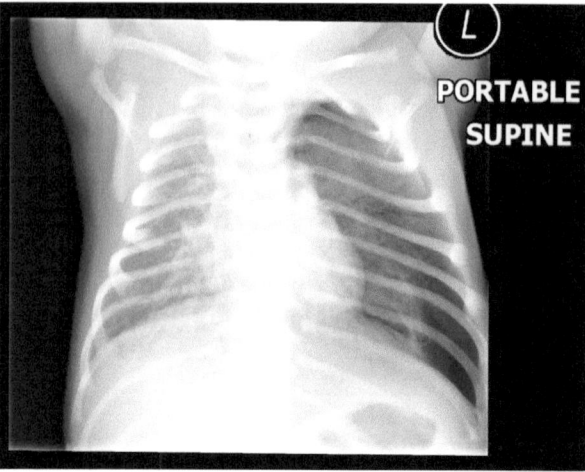

Figure 1.5 Anteroposterior chest image demonstrating rotation and a false appearance of a left-sided pneumothorax in a neonate.

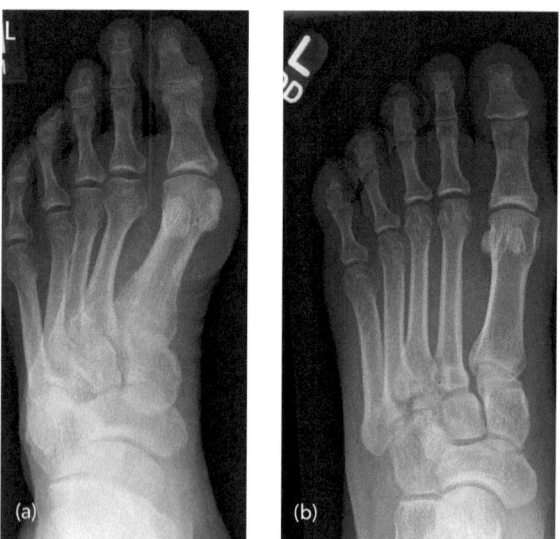

Figure 1.6 Anteroposterior foot images demonstrating (a) poor technique with the leg in external rotation and (b) good technique enabling visualisation of malalignment at the second tarsometatarsal joint and a third metatarsal fracture.

Some injuries may require additional projections to identify associated abnormalities. One injury pattern involves the '**ring bone**' or 'ring bone equivalent', the principle being that a ring cannot break in one place. A second injury (i.e. a fracture, dislocation/subluxation or diastasis) should be suspected if an injury is seen in the following locations:

- the main pelvic ring or the obturator rings of the pelvis;
- the facial bones – the mandible with skull and zygomatic arches;
- the ribs, sternum or spine;
- any vertebra or foramina transversaria in the cervical spine;
- the radius or ulna;
- the tibia or fibula.

Once it has been determined that the available images are adequate, the process of assessing the visible anatomy can begin.

Assessment of Bones

- The **cortex** of the bone should be smooth, and the bones should be of equal density. A fracture is generally a lucent line, but may be sclerotic if impaction has occurred.
- While trauma is the most common cause of abnormal bony appearances, a **pathological process** may also present as disruption in the cortex with or without a focal or patchy area of increased lucency or sclerosis. Some pathologies may need escalating to the referring clinician or expediting for a formal report, while there are some that can be ignored. Knowing the difference between the two will assist in recognising when escalation is required. Pathological processes are discussed in Section 6.
- Due to the bending coefficient of children's bones, they may not fracture when injured but **bend** or **buckle**. Additionally, evaluation of the metaphysis is important, as damage in this region can result in growth arrest. The effect of trauma on the developing bones is discussed in Chapter 2.

Assessment of Cartilaginous Areas

- The **articular surfaces** of opposing bones should be closely aligned with each other. Widening or malalignment may indicate dislocation, subluxation, diastasis or the presence of swelling within the joint, such as that caused by infection or an effusion, for example.

- **Diastasis** refers to the separation of two bones that are joined by ligaments, for example the distal tibia and fibula at the syndesmosis (**Figure 1.7a**).
- **Subluxation** is the partial malalignment of the joint with some contact remaining between the articular surfaces (**Figure 1.7b**). These can be subtle and are dependent on good technique.
- **Dislocation** is the complete malalignment of the bones forming the joint so that the articular surfaces are no longer in contact with each other (**Figure 1.7c**).

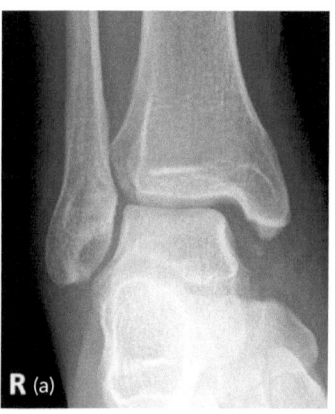 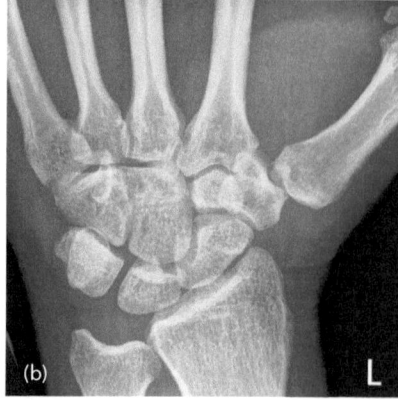

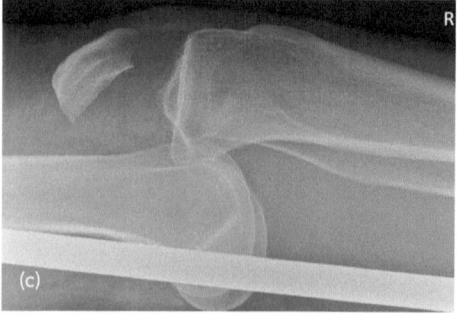

Figure 1.7
(a) Anteroposterior ankle image demonstrating distal tibiofibular diastasis. (b) Posteroanterior wrist image demonstrating first carpometacarpal subluxation. (c) Lateral knee image demonstrating tibiofemoral dislocation.

- **Joint spaces** may be reduced if there is a disease such as degenerative or rheumatoid arthritis. Although it may not need to be included within the comment, understanding joint disease will assist in excluding it as a finding requiring escalation. This will be outlined in Chapter 15.
- It is important to look for **fracture fragments** that could have moved into the joint space during reduction of a dislocation. These can lead to the joint not functioning correctly, giving way or locking.
- Irregularities within the **growth plate**, such as fragmentation, may indicate a non-displaced Salter–Harris injury, as discussed in Chapter 2.

Assessment of Soft Tissues

- The soft tissues should be **homogeneous**.
    - A lucency may be associated with a compound fracture or traumatic emphysema. In some instances, it may be gas within the soft tissues associated with infection.
    - A density may be associated with haematoma or soft tissue swelling. A focal area of increased density may indicate a retained foreign body, either acute or chronic.

- Increased fluid within the joint space can manifest as an **effusion** or a **lipohaemarthrosis (Figure 1.8)**. An effusion will have different characteristics depending on which joint is affected, and these will be discussed in the relevant chapters.

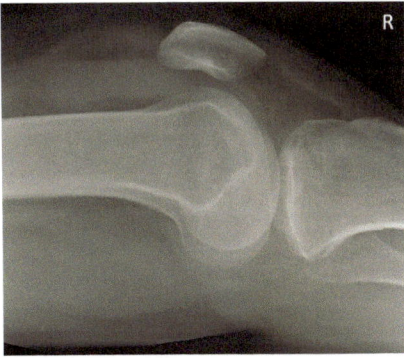

Figure 1.8 Lateral knee image demonstrating a lipohaemarthrosis.

- The soft tissues of the neck are key in identifying pathology involving the cervical spine, and these will be discussed in Chapter 11.
- The soft tissues of the chest and abdomen must always be evaluated if they are included on any images. These will be discussed in more detail in the relevant chapters.

Satisfaction of Search

Many abnormalities are easy to see, and this may cause the viewer to stop evaluating the image if they are satisfied that they have identified the answer to the clinical question. However, a second, sometimes more significant, abnormality may be overlooked if a systematic method is not followed. This is known as a '**satisfaction of search**' error. It is essential to continue reviewing the image until the process of evaluation is complete.

Figure 1.9 is an anteroposterior shoulder image of a patient presenting with shoulder pain. The patient is unclear about an injury but has a 'chronic alcohol use disorder', which has an impact on memory and the ability to think clearly. There is an acromioclavicular subluxation. Had the evaluation stopped at this point, the gas underneath the right diaphragm, indicating a perforation, may have been overlooked. Referred shoulder pain can precede the abdominal pain caused by a perforation. The collimation on this image is poor; however, the subdiaphragmatic area is visible and must be assessed.

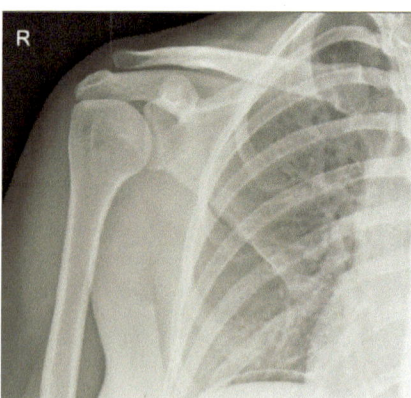

Figure 1.9 Anteroposterior shoulder image demonstrating a subluxed acromioclavicular joint and a perforation.

NORMAL VARIANTS

When evaluating images, a normal variant may be confused with a fracture or a pathology. There are a vast range of **normal variants**.[13] Of these, **accessory ossicles** may be confused with avulsion fractures. These are small, smooth, corticated fragments and are found in specific locations. Recognising these will enable this finding to be dismissed as an abnormality, but they can be a cause of pain[13] so, if the clinical history is simply that of pain, then the ossicle should be mentioned. The following will help differentiate between a fracture fragment and an accessory ossicle.

- Is there soft tissue swelling? This is more likely to be associated with a fracture.
- Is the cortex breached (i.e. is there an area within the adjacent bone from which the fragment may have originated)? If so, then it is a fracture.
- Has it got classical appearances of an accessory ossicle (i.e. small, smooth and corticated; **Figure 1.10**)?

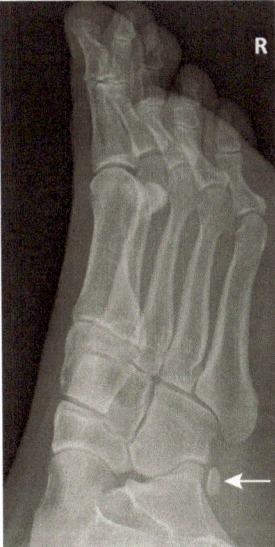

Figure 1.10 Accessory ossicle on a dorsi-plantar foot image.

- Is it in a typical position for an accessory ossicle? Refer to Keats and Anderson's *Atlas of Normal Roentgen Variants That May Simulate Disease*.[13]
- If this fragment was attached to the bone, would the bone take on an abnormal appearance? If so, it is more likely to be an accessory ossicle than a fracture fragment.

There are many additional normal variants in the paediatric skeleton, predominantly related to variations in the way that the bones develop. Many are associated with the epiphyses.

- **Multi-centre epiphyses** are created when the epiphysis develops not from one centre of ossification but from multiple centres of ossification, which eventually fuse together to form one epiphysis. These can occur anywhere in the growing skeleton, but one of the more common sites is the navicular (**Figure 1.11**).
- A **pseudo-epiphysis** is created when there is an attempt to create two epiphyses in a short bone. This will result in a cleft, which could be mistaken for a fracture (**Figure 1.11**).

Any apparent normal variant could be a pathology, and it is essential to interpret the appearances alongside the clinical presentation.

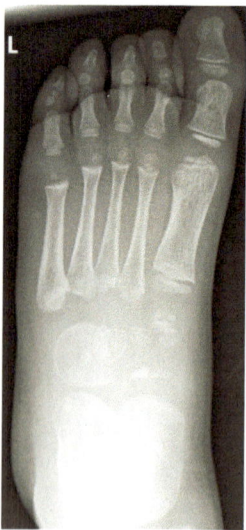

Figure 1.11 Dorsi-plantar foot image demonstrating multiple ossification centres for the navicular and medial cuneiform and a pseudo-epiphysis in the first metatarsal head and at the base of the third and fifth metatarsals.

CONSTRUCTING THE COMMENT

When the evaluation has been completed, the comment can be written. The clinical information must be reviewed again. As well as ensuring that the clinical question has been answered, if the abnormality does not correlate with the mechanism of injury or with the symptoms provided then the following should be considered:

- In vulnerable patients, the injury may be associated with **physical abuse**. The abnormality should be described with a suggestion that further clinical correlation occurs, and local safeguarding procedures must be followed. Section 5 will outline radiological signs of abuse.
- It may be an incidental finding of a normal variant.[13]

Radiographers are seen as the source of knowledge in relation to radiographic imaging, and their comment will add value to the patient pathway by assisting the referrer in the immediate management of their patient, so consideration needs to be given to the content. When abnormalities have been identified using the ABCs approach, the comment needs constructing to give as much detail as possible to the referring clinician. Following a template will allow a focused approach to this and result in a concise but informative comment (**Table 1.2**). This structured approach may differ depending on the abnormality and may need amending for complex cases, but starting off with a template will

Table 1.2 Template for developing a comment.

A	Abnormality type	Indicate the fracture, dislocation/subluxation or pathology.
B	Bone details	Identify the bones involved and be specific with the location of fractures.
C	Cartilage involvement	Include any involvement of the articular surface or growth plate.
D	Displacement	Explain the direction of any movement at the fracture site or malalignment of joints.
E	Extra features	Indicate if there are any other features that may be concerning.

help build confidence and the development of a commenting style. There are blank templates to support the evaluation of the image and the construction of the comment for use by readers in Table 1.4 at the end of the chapter.

Abnormality type. Comments are predominantly related to ED imaging, so fractures and dislocations will be the most common abnormalities seen. A simple comment, for example 'fractured radius', will tell the referrer the location of a fracture, but including the type of fracture will give the referrer more information from which to develop a management plan. 'Buckle fracture distal radius' indicates a stable injury that can be treated conservatively; however, 'comminuted fracture distal radius' suggests that early orthopaedic input is required.

Bone details. The location of a fracture should be indicated (e.g. midshaft or distal, epiphyseal or metaphyseal). **Figure 1.12** demonstrates gross bone anatomy.

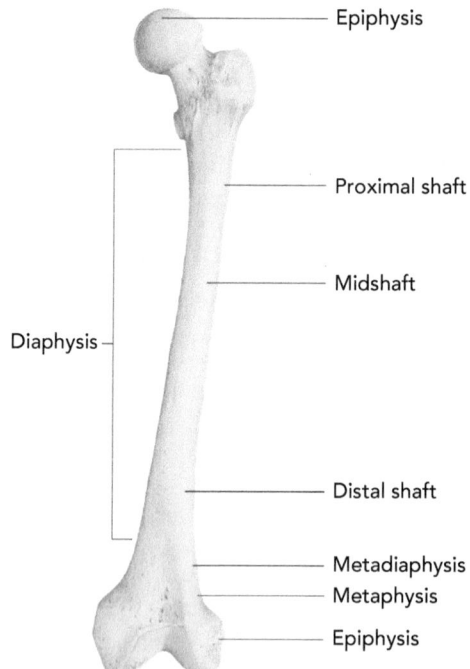

Epiphysis

Proximal shaft

Midshaft

Diaphysis

Distal shaft

Metadiaphysis
Metaphysis
Epiphysis

Figure 1.12 Gross anatomy of a long bone.

Cartilage involvement. The comment must include any involvement of a joint or growth plate.

Displacement. This describes the direction of movement at a fracture site or malalignment at a joint and is described in relation to the direction in which the distal part has moved. There are several ways of describing a fracture in which there has been movement at the fracture site:

- **displacement** – the fractured bone ends are not in contact with each other (**Figure 1.13a**);
- **angulation** – the fractured bone ends are in contact with each other, but the long axis of the bone is disrupted (**Figure 1.13b**);
- **distraction** – the gap between the fractured bone ends is widened but the long axis of the bone is generally maintained (**Figure 1.13c**);
- **rotation** – there is rotation of the distal part of the bone in relation to the long axis; adjacent joints need to be seen to accurately identify this (**Figure 1.13d**).

Extra features. There may be other features on the image that are worthy of comment, such as soft tissue signs, normal variants or pathologies.

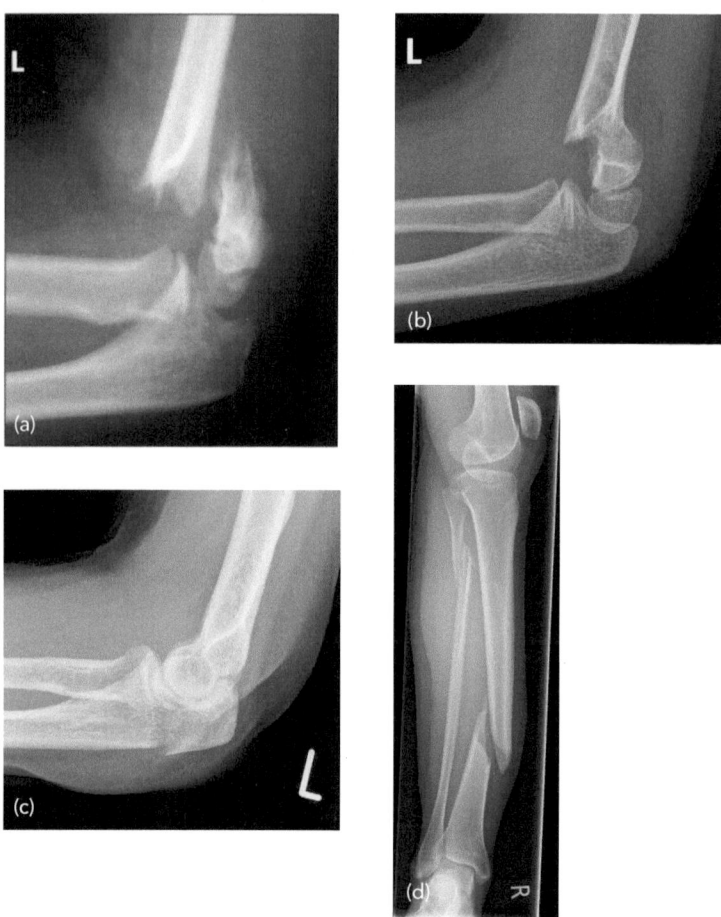

Figure 1.13 Lateral elbow images demonstrating (a) posterior displacement, (b) posterior angulation and (c) distraction. (d) Anteroposterior tibia and fibula image demonstrating lateral rotation.

CHAPTER SUMMARY

- The use of a standard method for evaluation should ensure the whole image is reviewed and any abnormality is detected. This is summarised in **Table 1.3**.
- When describing a fracture or joint malalignment, the direction of movement of the distal part must be described.
- Recognition of the wide range of normal variants will reduce commenting errors.
- Concerning features must be raised with the referring clinician.
- Commenting templates help in structuring the comment (**Table 1.4**).

Table 1.3 Summary of ABCs of evaluation.

Adequacy	Viewing conditions must be optimised.
	Correct projections must be obtained to demonstrate relevant anatomy.
	Images must be technically correct.
	Exposure factors must be selected to optimise image quality.
Bones	Cortices must be smooth with no breaks or buckles.
	Bones should be of equal density with no lucent or sclerotic areas.
Cartilaginous areas	Articular surfaces of opposing bones should be aligned.
	There should be no irregularities within the growth plate.
	Joint spaces should not be widened or reduced.
	Joint spaces should be clear with no bone fragments or calcifications visible.
Soft tissues	These should be homogeneous with no areas of lucency or increwased density.
	Soft tissues around the joints may demonstrate an effusion or a lipohaemarthrosis.
	Chest/abdominal soft tissues should be assessed if they are included on the image.
Satisfaction of search	Make sure that a complete evaluation of the image has taken place using the above search strategy.

Table 1.4 Templates for developing a comment.

Thought process following the ABCs systematic method of evaluation	
Adequacy	_____
Bones	_____
Cartilaginous areas	_____
Soft tissues	_____
Satisfaction of search	_____

Developing the comment		
A	Abnormality type	_____
B	Bone details	_____
C	Cartilage involvement	_____
D	Displacement	_____
E	Extra features	_____

Writing the comment
Add your comment text here.

_____

_____

_____

REFERENCES

1. Price, R. Critical factors influencing the changing scope of practice; the defining periods. *Imaging and Oncology* 2005;6–11.
2. Renwick, I.G.H., Burt, W.P. and Stelle, B. How well can radiographers triage X-ray films in accident and emergency departments? *British Medical Journal* 1991;**302**:568–569.
3. Saxton, H.M. Should radiologists report on every film? *Clinical Radiology* 1992;**45**:1–3.
4. Loughran, C.F. Reporting of fracture radiographs by radiographers – the impact of a training programme. *British Journal of Radiology* 1994;**67**:945–950
5. Berman, L., de Lacey, G., Twomey, E., Twomey, B., Welch, T. and Eban, R. Reducing errors in accident department; a simple method using radiographers. *British Medical Journal* 1985;**290**:421–422.
6. Audit Commission. *Improving Your Image – How to Manage Radiology Services More Effectively.* London: HMSO, 1995.
7. Royal College of Radiologists. *Medical Staffing and Workload in Clinical Radiology in the United Kingdom.* London: Royal College of Radiologists, 1993.
8. College of Radiographers. *Code of Professional Conduct.* London: College of Radiographers, 1993.
9. College of Radiographers. *Medical Image Interpretation and Clinical Reporting by Non-radiologists: The Role of the Radiographer.* London: College of Radiographers, 2006.
10. Beardmore, C. *Preliminary Clinical Evaluation and Clinical Reporting by Radiographers: Policy and Practice Guidance.* London: College of Radiographers, 2013.
11. HM Government. *The Ionising Radiation (Medical Exposure) Regulations.* London: The Stationery Office, 2017.
12. Nicholson, D.A. and Driscoll, P. *ABC of Emergency Radiology*, ABC Series. Hoboken, NJ: Wiley-Blackwell, 1995.
13. Keats, T.E. and Anderson, M.W. *Atlas of Normal Roentgen Variants That May Simulate Disease*, 9th edn. Philadelphia, PA: Saunders, 2012.

2. BONE PHYSIOLOGY

Accurate image evaluation requires a good understanding of detailed bony anatomy, but evaluation errors may also be made if there is poor knowledge of the physiological processes of bone. Due to the way that the skeleton develops, matures and ages, different injury patterns may be seen with similar mechanisms of injury. For example, a fall onto the outstretched hand (FOOSH) is the most common mechanism of injury, and the forces can be absorbed anywhere from the wrist to the clavicle, resulting in a fracture or dislocation at any point in the upper limb and shoulder girdle. An adult is more likely to sustain a complete fracture (**Figure 2.1a**), while a child's bones may buckle (**Figure 2.1b**) or bend. Additionally, fractures involving the growth plates will be seen in the immature skeleton, while reduced bone density in the older population can result in fragility fractures. No matter the age of the patient, the stages of fracture healing are the same, albeit bones heal faster in children.

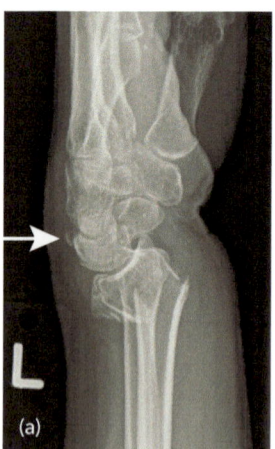 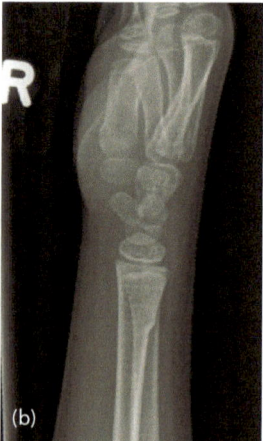

Figure 2.1 Lateral wrist images obtained following FOOSH and demonstrating (a) a transverse radial fracture in an adult with an avulsion fracture from the triquetral (white arrow) and (b) a dorsal radial buckle fracture in a child.

BONE DEVELOPMENT AND GROWTH

Around 6 weeks after conception, the skeletal cartilaginous model is fully developed but not ossified. Once ossification begins, it is either intramembranous or enchondral. The flat bones of the skull and facial bones are examples of **intramembranous ossification**, in which mesenchymal cells convert into osteoblasts, which secrete osteoid. This calcifies and traps osteoblasts, which convert into osteocytes. Additional osteoblasts develop around the periphery of the calcified matrix, and the bone continues to grow in this way until skeletal maturation.

Long and short bones develop through **enchondral ossification** (**Figure 2.2**). In these bones, the mesenchymal cells change into chondrocytes, which help shape the cartilaginous model. The chondrocytes die, leaving a cavitated matrix, which becomes the frame for the developing bone. Blood vessel infiltration results in a primary ossification centre in the middle of the cartilaginous model 2 to 4 months after conception. This becomes the diaphysis. Further vessels infiltrate the ends of the model, resulting in a secondary ossification centre, also known as an epiphysis. Long bones have two epiphyses, while short bones have only one. Some epiphyses are present at birth, but others do not appear until the late teens. The age of appearance and rate of growth is specific to that bone, enabling an assessment of bone maturity known as bone ageing and performed when a child is growing slower or faster than expected for their age.

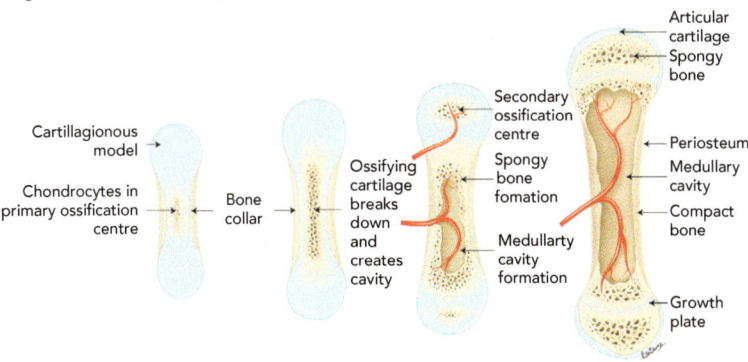

Figure 2.2 Enchondral ossification.

The epiphyses grow until the cartilaginous model is replaced with bone. Growth in length occurs at the physis, or **growth plate**, which is between the diaphysis and the epiphysis. There are four levels of cells within each growth plate (**Figure 2.3**).

1. **Zone of resting cartilage.** This is adjacent to the epiphysis and made up of chondrocytes, which are inactive. They are disorganised and surrounded by a large amount of extracellular matrix.
2. **Zone of proliferating cartilage.** The chondrocytes become active, divide and form columns.
3. **Zone of maturing cartilage.** The chondrocytes grow, and the columns extend towards the metaphysis.
4. **Zone of calcifying cartilage.** Minerals are deposited within the matrix formed by the chondrocytes adjacent to the metaphysis. Calcification starts and the chondrocytes die, as they are unable to receive nutrients from the calcifying matrix. This zone is the weakest part of the immature skeleton, as it has not developed the strength of mature bone and is most likely to be damaged following injury.

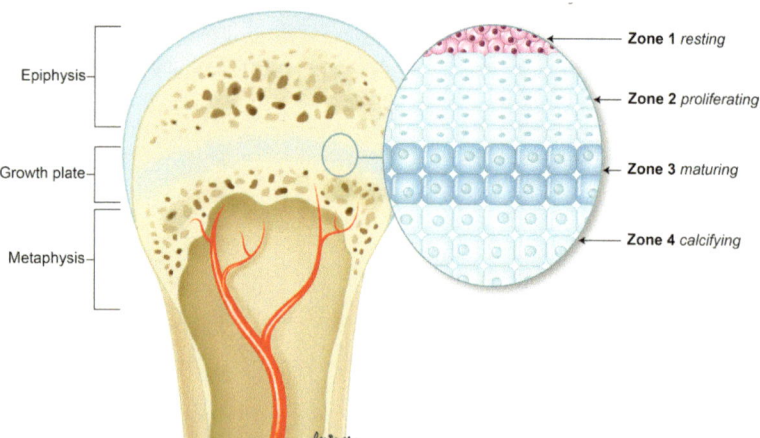

Figure 2.3 Zones within the growth plate.

Any injury involving the growth plate is classified according to its relationship with the epiphysis, growth plate and metaphysis using the Salter–Harris (SH) classification. They are:

- **SHI** (SH type I). The fracture is through the zone of calcifying cartilage without extension into the metaphysis or epiphysis. It may appear as widening of the growth plate or a slip of the epiphysis (**Figure 2.4a**). This type of fracture rarely causes complications.
- **SHII.** The fracture is through the zone of calcifying cartilage, and it extends into the metaphysis (**Figure 2.4b**). This is the most common of all the SH-type injuries and rarely causes complications, despite sometimes looking significantly displaced.
- **SHIII.** The fracture is through the zone of calcifying cartilage extending through the epiphysis to the articular surface (**Figure 2.4c**), making it an intra-articular fracture. The zone of proliferating cartilage is damaged, and this may lead to growth complications, depending on the bone involved and the age of the patient. Complications will not be as noticeable if the fracture occurs close to skeletal maturation, but if this occurs in a young child who has still got substantive growth to take place, then any disruption to that growth is likely to cause structural deformity.
- **SHIV.** The fracture extends from the articular cartilage, through the growth plate and into the metaphysis (**Figure 2.4d**). It may need two projections to be able to see both components of the fracture. As the zone of proliferating cartilage has been breached, growth complications can occur, again dependent on the bone involved and the age of the child. This is also an intra-articular fracture.
- **SHV.** This is an exceedingly rare injury and not diagnosed at initial presentation. It involves segmental crushing of the growth plate, which damages the zone of proliferating cartilage and causes consequent growth disturbance, usually identified on later images by early fusion at the growth plate.

Growth in width occurs when cells within the perichondrium, a layer of connective tissue covering the cartilaginous model, convert into osteoblasts and surround the model with a collar of bone. The skeleton stops growing around 18 years in females and 20 years in males, although ossification continues in some bones until around 25 years, with the clavicle being the last bone to stop growing.

Also present in children's bones is an apophysis (discussed in relevant chapters). This does not contribute to growth unless it is found on an irregular or flat bone where it contributes to circumferential growth. Its main purpose is for tendon connection, and it can become avulsed.

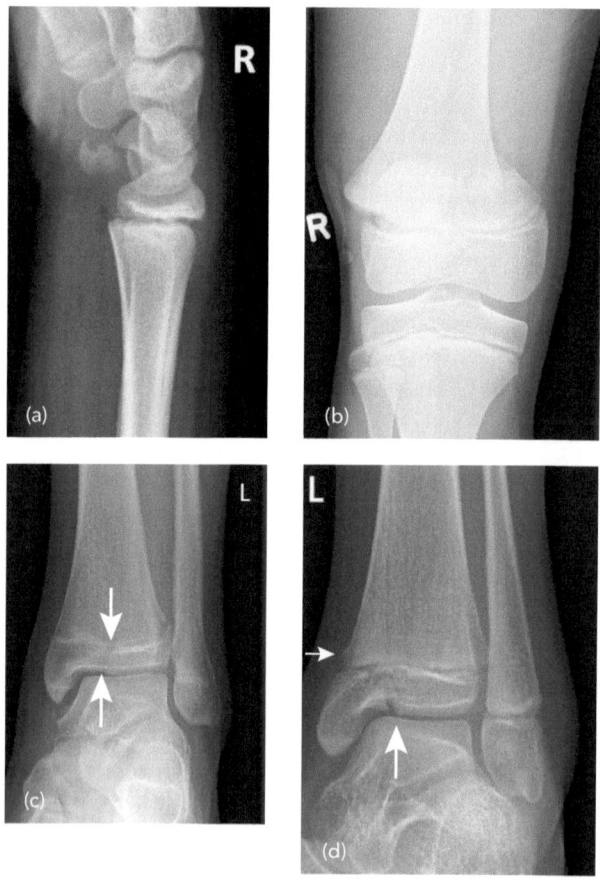

Figure 2.4 (a) Lateral wrist image demonstrating an SHI injury. (b) Anteroposterior knee image demonstrating an SHII injury. (c) Anteroposterior ankle image demonstrating an SHIII injury. (d) Anteroposterior ankle image demonstrating an SHIV injury.

DECLINE IN BONE HEALTH

There is a global increase in the older population, with old age being defined as over 65 years.[1] With old age and some illnesses in younger patients, there is a decline in bone health, which leads to osteoporosis, a progressive bone disease in which osteoclasts work faster than osteoblasts, changing the mineral make-up of the bone and negatively affecting bone density. Although this cannot be quantified on the plain X-ray image, thinned cortices and increased radiolucency are visible (**Figure 2.5**). This is referred to radiologically as **osteopenia**. It is this loss in bone mass that leads to insufficiency fractures commonly seen in the spine and hip. There is also a decline in physical and mental health, with this having a further impact on the risk of falls and associated injury in older people.[2] These patients tend to have a range of comorbidities and, when involved in trauma, they are managed on a **Silver Trauma** pathway,[3] which considers the multiple factors that have an impact on and possibly elevate an initial innocuous low-level injury into major trauma with significant adverse outcomes.[4] One area of concern is rib fractures, in relation to which pulmonary complications such as pneumonia are twice as likely in older people, with the mortality rate increasing with the number of ribs fractured.[5]

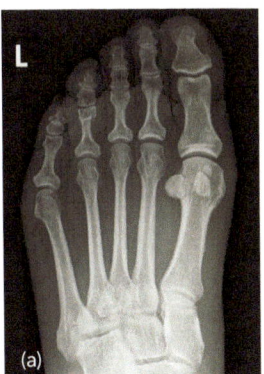
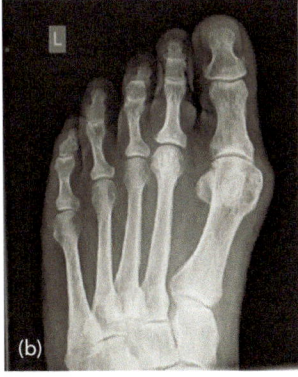

Figure 2.5 Dorsi-palmar foot images demonstrating (a) normal cortical thickness in a young healthy patient and (b) thinned cortices (compare the metatarsal shafts) in a patient with low bone density.

FRACTURE HEALING

Bone is highly vascular and constantly remodelling, with osteoclasts clearing bone and osteoblasts building bone. Due to the enhanced activity in the growing skeleton, fractures in children heal quickly and remodel, leaving little sign of injury. Fracture healing slows down with age due to the reduced level of bone metabolism.

There are four stages to fracture healing.

1. **Stage 1: inflammation.** This initial stage commences immediately after the initial insult to the bone. It involves the formation of a haematoma containing fibroblasts, which convert to chondroblasts and form granulation tissue. This granulation tissue bridges the fracture (**Figure 2.6a**), taking up to 5 days in a child and 2 weeks in an adult.
2. **Stage 2: soft callus.** Resorption around the fracture site widens the fracture line, and osteoblastic activity causes a **periosteal reaction**, which will be visible on the image. Cells within the granulation tissue convert into fibroblasts and chondroblasts and this is a soft callus (**Figure 2.6b**). This takes up to 3 weeks in a child and 6 weeks in an adult.
3. **Stage 3: hard callus.** The soft callus converts into a hard callus through a process such as enchondral ossification and the fracture line starts to blur (**Figure 2.6c**). This takes up to 6 weeks in a child and 6 months in an adult.
4. **Stage 4: remodelling.** This final stage can take up to 3 months in a child and 2 years in an adult and involves the bone attempting to return to its original templated shape. The fracture line is almost invisible on images (**Figure 2.6d**).

Understanding this process will help in identifying fractures that may be at risk of non-union, usually diagnosed if there is no evidence of healing after 9 months or if the process stops for 3 months before completion of healing. This is demonstrated by a persistent fracture line with fracture margins having a sclerotic appearance. Fracture healing in a healthy patient may be affected by the level of comminution, displacement or soft tissue damage, infection from the initial injury or

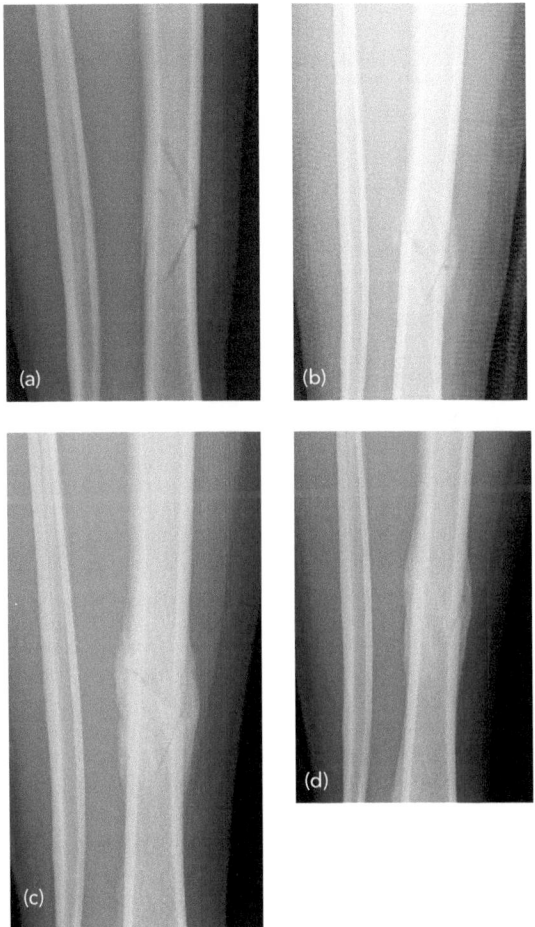

Figure 2.6 The stages of fracture healing: (a) inflammation, (b) soft callus, (c) hard callus and (d) remodelling.

surgical intervention. It may also be affected by smoking, alcohol intake and low levels of vitamins and minerals, in particular vitamins C and D and calcium. Additionally, understanding the fracture healing process will help in being able to estimate when a fracture occurred, which is an important aspect of imaging in suspected physical abuse.

CHAPTER SUMMARY

- It is essential that there is a good underpinning knowledge of anatomy and physiology.
- Recognition of bone development and growth will aid in interpreting the often-confusing appearance of children's images.
- The weakest part of the skeleton of a child is the newly calcified bone adjacent to the metaphysis, so the forces from an injury are more likely to be absorbed in this area.
- Understanding the ageing process of bone will help identify appearances of osteopenia and associated fractures caused by reduction in bone density.
- Knowledge of stages of fracture healing is imperative in identifying abusive signs.

REFERENCES

1. Age UK. *Later Life in the United Kingdom*. London: Age UK, 2019.
2. Hollinghurst, R., Williams, N., Pedrick-Case, R., North, L., Long, S., Fry, R. et al. Annual risk of falls resulting in emergency department and hospital attendances for older people: an observational study of 781,081 individuals living in Wales (United Kingdom) including deprivation, frailty and dementia diagnosis between 2010 and 2020. *Age and Ageing* 2022;**51**(8):afac176.
3. Conroy, S. *Silver Book II: Quality Care for Older People with Urgent Care Needs*. London: British Geriatrics Society, 2021.
4. Hendrickson, S.A., Osei-Kuffour, D., Aylwin, C., Fertleman, M. and Hettiaratchy, S. 'Silver' trauma: predicting mortality in elderly major trauma based on place of injury. *Scandinavian Journal of Trauma, Resuscitation and Emergency* 2015;**23**(Suppl 2):A4.
5. Witt, C.E. and Bulgar, E.M. Comprehensive approach to the management of the patient with multiple rib fractures: a review and introduction of a bundled rib fracture management protocol. *Trauma Surgery and Acute Care Open* 2017;**2**(1):e000064.

SECTION 2
UPPER LIMB TRAUMA

3. HAND AND WRIST

There are many bones and joints to evaluate in the hand and wrist and many ways of doing this, whether by moving distally from the wrist or proximally from the fingers, for example. Consistency in the approach will result in a more accurate and speedy evaluation process.

One of the more common mechanisms of injury across all ages is a fall onto the outstretched hand (**FOOSH**) resulting in fractures involving the distal radius and ulna. Additionally, young adults have sporting or fighting injuries and young children sustain crush injuries from entrapment in doors. **Table 3.1** summarises these injuries and the resultant abnormalities.

Table 3.1 Common mechanisms of injury and associated abnormalities in the hand and wrist.

Mechanism	Typical abnormality
Crush injury	Comminuted fracture of the distal phalanx Transverse fracture of the phalanges or MCs
Hyperflexion or hyperextension injuries	Fracture to the base of the proximal phalanx; may manifest as an SHII fracture in children Avulsion fracture from the base of the distal or middle phalanx Interphalangeal joint subluxation or dislocation Fracture to the base of the first MC
Axial compression/ punch injury	SHV fracture in children Fracture of the MC neck, commonly the fifth MC Hamate fracture
Direct blow	Transverse radius/ulna fracture
FOOSH	Fracture of the radius/ulna (any age) Buckle fracture of the radius/ulna (4–10 years) SHII fracture to the distal radius (11–16 years) Scaphoid or triquetral fracture (above 12 years) Lunate or perilunate dislocation

MC, metacarpal; SH(I, II, etc.), Salter–Harris type (I, II, etc.).

Building on the ABCs method of evaluation, as introduced in Chapter 1, and assuming that adequacy has been checked, **Table 3.2** describes the checks unique to the evaluation of hand and wrist images. **Figures 3.1a** and **b** demonstrate normal appearances on a dorsi-palmar (DP) hand image and a lateral wrist image, respectively, summarising these additional checks for hand and wrist images, which will be discussed in more detail in this chapter.

Table 3.2 Summary of the ABCs method of evaluation for the hand and wrist.

Focus	Points to consider
Bones	Cortices must be smooth with no breaks or buckles; in particular, the metaphyseal region of a child's bones must be carefully inspected.
	The zone of vulnerability must be assessed carefully if a single injury is seen within this zone.
	Each carpal bone must be identified by name so that a fractured bone is not mistaken for two carpal bones.
Cartilaginous areas	On the DP image, the carpal arcs must be demonstrated as smooth virtual curves.
	On the lateral image, there should be clear alignment through the third metacarpal, the capitate and lunate, and the distal radius.
	Intercarpal joint spaces should be no more than 2 mm in the skeletally mature patient.
	The distal radio-ulna alignment must be maintained. If it is disrupted, there may be a breach in the 'ring bone'.
Soft tissues	On the DP image, the scaphoid fat stripe, if visible, must lie in close relation to the scaphoid.
	On the lateral wrist image, the pronator quadratus fat stripe must lie in close relation to the distal radius.

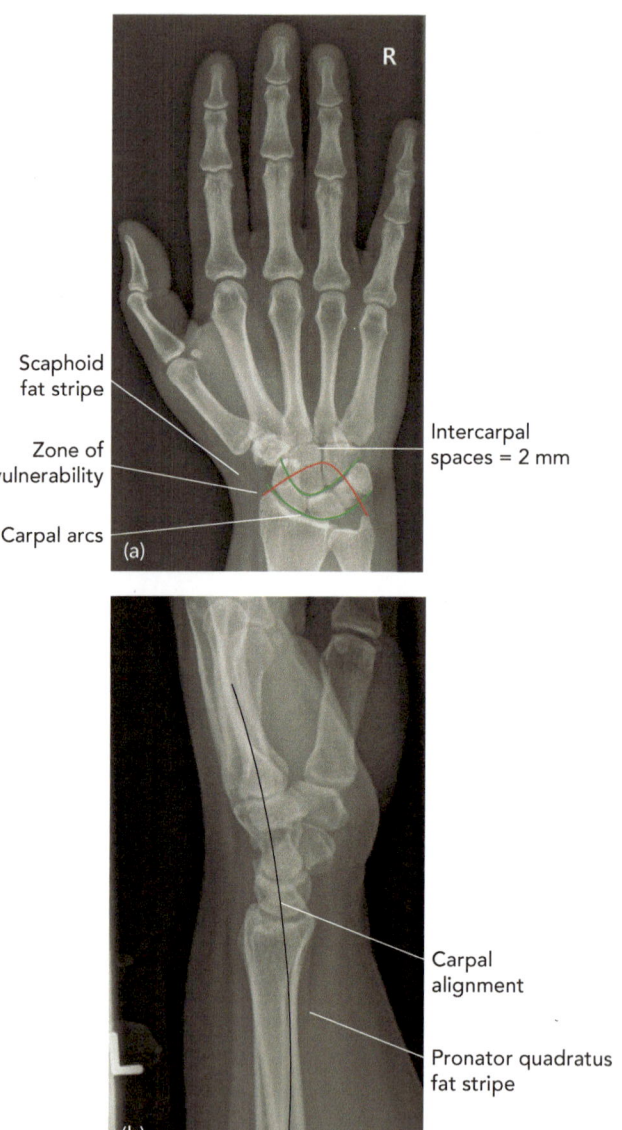

Scaphoid
fat stripe

Zone of
vulnerability

Carpal arcs

(a)

Intercarpal
spaces = 2 mm

Carpal
alignment

Pronator quadratus
fat stripe

(b)

Figure 3.1 (a) DP hand and (b) lateral wrist images demonstrating the checks that are unique to this area.

BONES

- Careful assessment should be made at the bases of the phalanges, as hyperflexion and hyperextension injuries may result in small fractures, the diagnosis of which is reliant on a good lateral image of the finger and will not be seen on an oblique image such as that obtained when doing an oblique hand X-ray.

  - Hyperflexion causes either a distal interphalangeal joint (DIPJ) injury known as a **mallet deformity** or a proximal interphalangeal joint (PIPJ) injury known as a **boutonniere deformity**. While there is rarely a fracture associated with the latter, a small avulsion fracture from the dorsal base of the distal phalanx may be visible in a mallet deformity (**Figure 3.2a**).
  - Hyperextension causes the volar plate ligament to avulse a small fragment from the palmar base of the middle phalanx, called a **volar plate fracture (Figure 3.2b)**. If the fragment is large, there may be a dorsal subluxation or dislocation at the PIPJ.

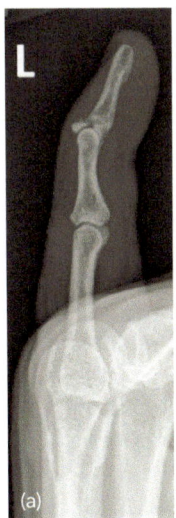
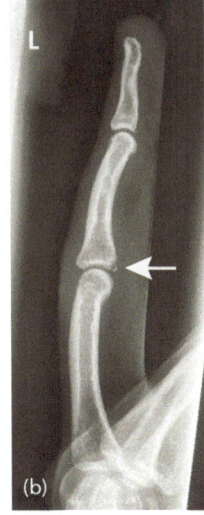

Figure 3.2 Lateral finger images demonstrating (a) a hypeflexion mallet deformity to the DIPJ and (b) a hyperextension avulsion fracture from the middle phalanx.

- Until skeletal maturity, at which point the metaphysis and epiphysis fuse, the weakest part of the skeleton is the newly calcified bone adjacent to the metaphysis. Hyperextension may result in a fracture in this region of the proximal phalanx, which commonly extends to the growth plate in a **Salter–Harris (SH) II** injury (**Figure 3.3**) and can be very subtle.

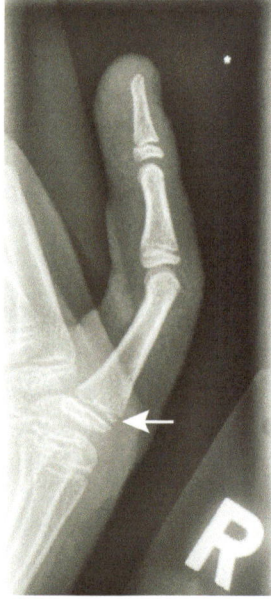

Figure 3.3 Lateral finger image demonstrating an SHII injury of the proximal phalanx.

- A fracture through the neck of the fifth metacarpal (MC) is caused by a force to the clenched hand and is commonly known as a **boxer's fracture**. While this is a classical appearance, there are also other fractures caused by the same mechanism of injury: a fracture through the base of the fourth MC and a fracture of the hamate. **Figure 3.4** demonstrates the need for three images to be able to see all components of this injury. A fourth MC fracture can be seen on the DP image, and a hamate fracture can be seen on the oblique image, but is better seen on the lateral image as a large fragment on the dorsum of the carpus.

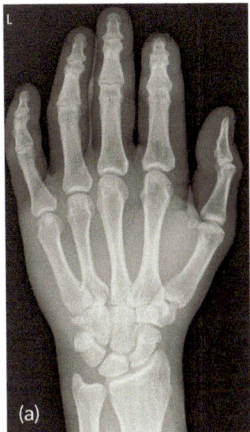 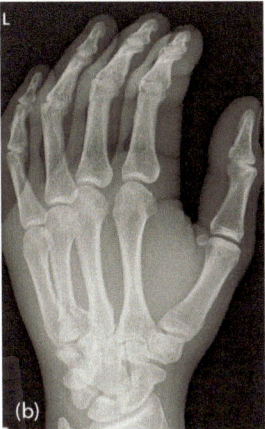 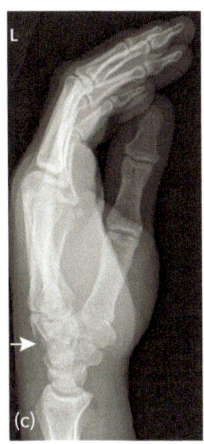

Figure 3.4 (a) DP, (b) DP oblique and (c) lateral hand images demonstrating multiple fractures (arrows) caused by a punch injury.

Comment: fractures through the base of the fourth MC and the hamate.

- Within the carpal bones, the most common fracture is a **scaphoid fracture** with the mechanism of injury being FOOSH. Fractures generally occur in the scaphoid waist, and 90% heal without problems if identified and treated correctly (**Figure 3.5a**).[1] A scaphoid fracture lies within the **zone of vulnerability**, which is an arc passing from the radial styloid process to the ulna styloid process (Figure 3.1a). If a fracture is identified within the zone of vulnerability, other fractures may be present within this zone and a computed tomography (CT) scan may be performed for full evaluation of the injury. Scaphoid fractures are at risk of non-union, and those within the proximal pole may develop osteonecrosis due to interruption of the blood supply. Non-union is identified as a fracture that is still visible 9 months after the initial injury and no progression of healing within the previous 3 months. Sclerosis is usually seen at the fracture margins in non-union cases (**Figure 3.5b**).
- Although carpal fractures are rare under the age of 12 years due to the amount of residual cartilage, scaphoid fractures in older children tend to involve the distal pole.

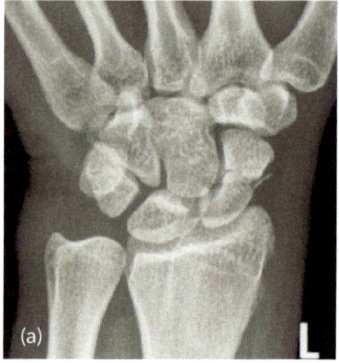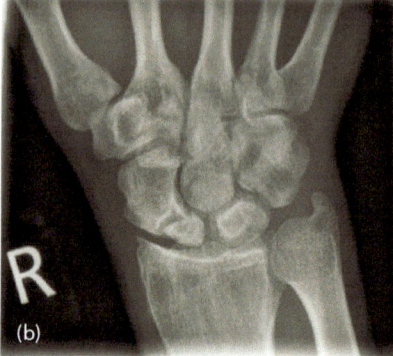

Figure 3.5 DP wrist images demonstrating (a) a scaphoid fracture within the zone of vulnerability and (b) non-union of a fracture through the proximal pole of the scaphoid.

- A **triquetral fracture** is the second most common carpal bone fracture. The mechanism of injury is impact to the dorsum of the hand and this type of fracture may be seen only on the lateral wrist image (Figure 2.1a). The appearance on an X-ray image is subtle, and a bone fragment in the soft tissues with soft tissue swelling and an appropriate mechanism of injury should help in identifying this fracture and differentiating it from the os epilunatum, an accessory ossicle lying proximal to the triquetral.
- While **distal radius and ulna fractures** are generally easy to see in adults, with **Colles fractures** being common in older patients (**Figure 3.6**), they can be subtle in children, so careful assessment of the cortex is needed, looking for deviation from the normally smooth contour. **Buckle fractures** are usually on the dorsal cortex as in Figure 2.1b, but can also occur in the anterior cortex (**Figure 3.7a**). A **greenstick fracture** is an incomplete fracture that breaches one cortex and then branches out within the medullary cavity not reaching the opposite cortex (**Figure 3.7b**). Fractures in the metaphyseal region may extend to the growth plate, with SHII injuries being the most common distal radius fracture in children (**Figure 3.7c**).

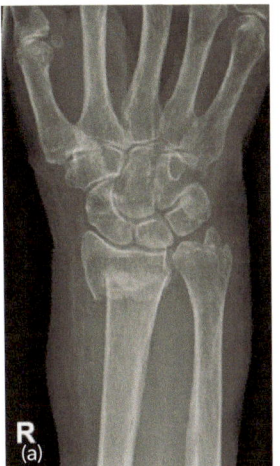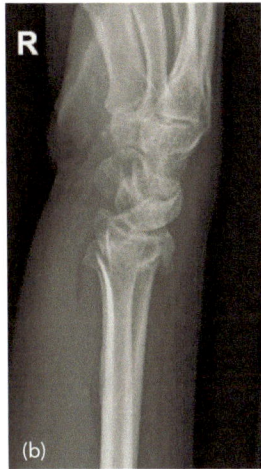

Figure 3.6 (a) DP and (b) lateral wrist images demonstrating a Colles fracture.

Comment: dorsally angulated fracture through the distal radius and avulsion of the ulna styloid process.

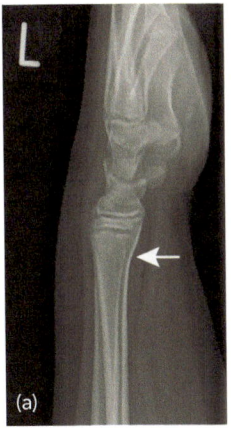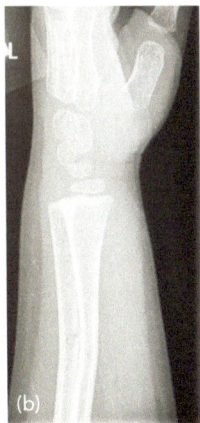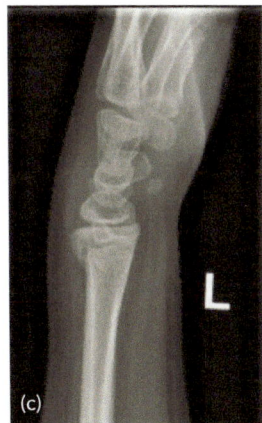

Figure 3.7 Lateral wrist images demonstrating distal radius fractures: (a) anterior buckle, (b) greenstick (also involving the ulna) and (c) SHII distal radius.

CARTILAGINOUS AREAS

- Joint spaces should be seen clearly. Flexion can cause superimposition of the bones either side of the joint, but this will also be seen at adjacent joints if this is a positional error. If there is superimposition at only one joint as in **Figure 3.8**, this suggests a **subluxation or dislocation**. A lateral hand image is needed for full evaluation.

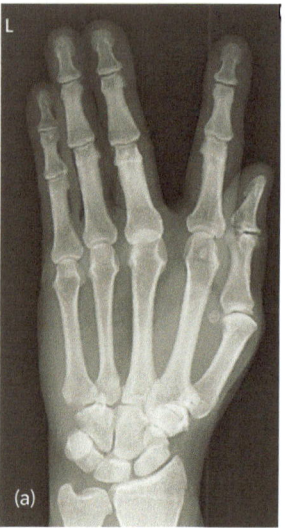 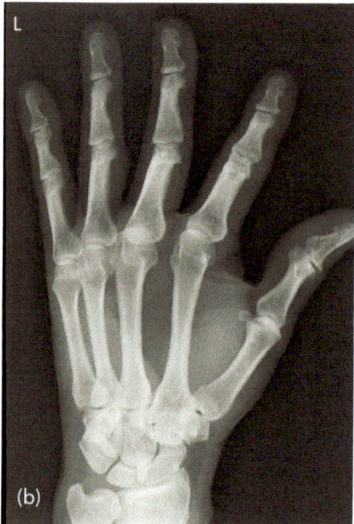

Figure 3.8 (a) DP and (b) DP oblique hand images demonstrating malalignment at the third metacarpophalangeal joint.

> **Comment: anterior displacement at the third metacarpophalangeal joint.**

- On the DP image, the carpal arcs should be seen as smooth curves connecting the proximal articular margins of the distal and proximal rows of the carpal bones (Figure 3.1a). Any disruption in the curve may indicate a fracture, subluxation or dislocation of a carpal bone, although these are less reliable in children when the carpus is not fully developed.

■ The spaces between the carpal bones should not exceed 2 mm in a skeletally mature hand. Widening of the joint spaces may indicate dislocation or ligamentous injury, more commonly between the scaphoid and lunate in an injury called a **scapho-lunate disassociation (Figure 3.9a).**

■ Reduction in a joint space may be caused by degenerative disease, which is commonly seen at the first carpometacarpal joint (CMCJ) and the triscaphe joint (**Figure 3.9b**).

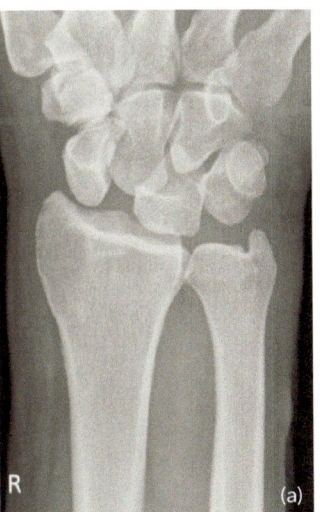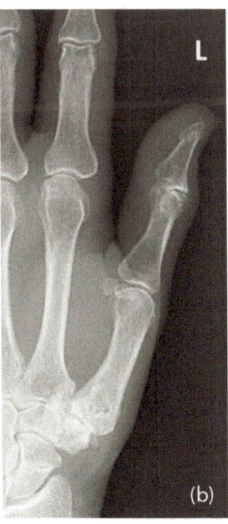

Figure 3.9 Images demonstrating disruption at the cartilaginous areas with (a) widening at the scapho-lunate junction and (b) reduction caused by degeneration at the first CMCJ and triscaphe joint.

■ On the lateral image, the lunate and capitate should be in alignment with the distal radius proximally and the third MC distally (Figure 3.1b). This is the carpal alignment line and is an indicator for displacement of a carpal bone, most commonly the lunate in a **lunate dislocation**. The lunate rotates and dislocates anteriorly, and the capitate moves proximally into the gap (**Figure 3.10a**). Although this is a rare injury, it is important that it is identified and treated without delay due to the neurological complications and ligamentous ruptures associated with it. This disruption may be associated with other injuries within the zone of vulnerability.

- A lunate dislocation must be differentiated from a **perilunate dislocation**, caused by dorsiflexion with radial or ulna deviation, in which the lunate stays in position, but the remainder of the carpus moves dorsally and sits behind the carpal alignment line (**Figure 3.10b**). Between 16% and 25% of perilunate injuries are missed at first presentation.[2] These injuries have an impact on the zone of vulnerability and the patient is likely to require a CT scan to fully evaluate the complexities of this injury pattern.

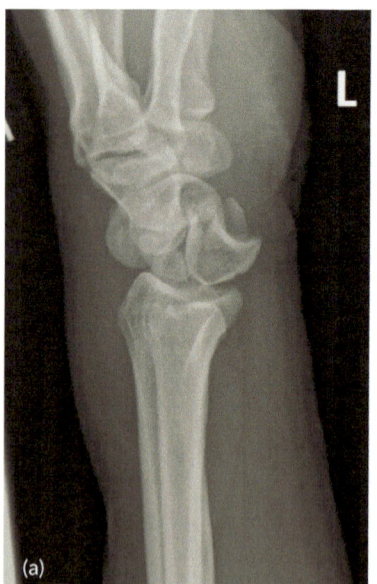
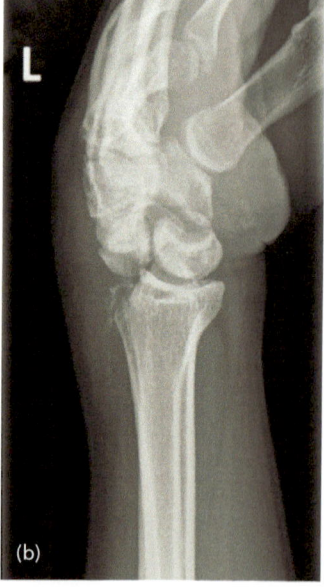

Figure 3.10 Lateral wrist images demonstrating (a) lunate dislocation and (b) perilunate dislocation with a fracture through the dorsal cortex of the distal radius.

SOFT TISSUES

- The **scaphoid fat stripe** is seen as an increased lucency on the lateral aspect of the scaphoid, where a small fat pad sits between the radial collateral ligament and the tendon sheaths (Figure 3.1a). Elevation of the fat stripe may indicate a scaphoid fracture due to increased fluid within the joint capsule. The normal fat stripe has a concavity, while the elevated fat stripe is convex. Some studies show it not to be a reliable sign;[3] however, it may help support an ambiguous appearance.
- The normal **pronator quadratus fat stripe**, associated with the pronator quadratus muscle, lies along the anterior surface of the distal radius (Figure 3.1b). If there is bleeding from a subtle fracture, this may be displaced away from the radius (**Figure 3.11**). As with the scaphoid fat stripe, some studies show it not to be a reliable sign,[3] but it may help support an equivocal finding in the distal radius. It is useful in supporting a diagnosis in children's injuries, such as subtle buckle fractures or undisplaced SHI injuries.

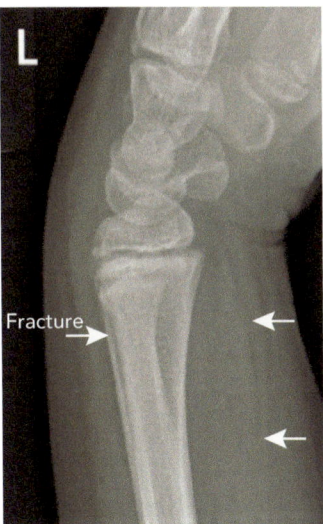

Figure 3.11 Lateral wrist image demonstrating elevation of the pronator quadratus fat pad with a buckle fracture in the dorsal cortex of the distal radius.

CHAPTER SUMMARY

- Children may have subtle fractures due to the composition of the bone, so the cortices must be carefully assessed to identify these fractures.
- Children's fractures may be closely associated with the metaphysis, so a check needs to be undertaken for lucencies next to the growth plate.
- A fracture in the zone of vulnerability should prompt close inspection of other bones and joint spaces within this zone.
- Close attention should be paid to the dorsum of the hand, looking for a small fragment that may be a triquetral fracture.
- The intercarpal joint spaces must be less than 2 mm in the skeletally mature patient. If greater than this, then there may be carpal instability caused by degeneration or injury.
- Soft tissue changes may be the only indication of injury. Elevation of fascial planes should be checked for, such as that of the pronator quadratus fat stripe.

REFERENCES

1. Winston, M.J. and Weiland, A.J. Scaphoid fractures in athletes. *Current Reviews in Musculoskeletal Medicine* 2017;**10**(1):38–44.
2. Navaratnam, A.V., Ball, S., Emerson, C. and Eckersley, R. Perilunate dislocation. *British Medical Journal* 2012;**345**:e7026.
3. Annamalai, G. and Raby, N. Scaphoid and pronator fat stripes are unreliable soft tissue signs in the detection of radiographically occult fractures. *Clinical Radiology* 2008;**58**(10):798–800.

4. RADIUS AND ULNA

Midshaft radius and ulna fractures are not usually difficult to see, as they are often displaced or angulated. Common mechanisms of injury include falls or direct blows (**Table 4.1**). However, isolated ulna fractures may be a reason to suspect abuse, as they can be caused when the arm is raised to prevent an impact to the face.

Table 4.1 Common mechanisms of injury and associated abnormalities in the radius and ulna.

Mechanism	Typical abnormality
Direct blow	Isolated fracture to ulna in defence injury
	Isolated fracture to radius
	Transverse fractures to radius and ulna
Fall	Fracture to midshaft of radius and ulna
	Fracture to radial head or neck (see Chapter 6 for further guidance)
	Plastic bowing fracture of radius and/or ulna

The radius and ulna configuration is classified as a **ring bone equivalent**. That means that the radius and ulna must be treated as a continuous ring and, if breached, a potential second injury must be sought (see Chapter 2 for further detail). When an isolated fracture of the midshaft of the radius or ulna is identified, it is important to assess the alignment of the adjacent joints to exclude an associated dislocation or subluxation. If the fracture occurs in the distal third of the radius or ulna, the second injury is commonly a tearing of the interosseous membrane, leading to an indiscernible widening of the distal radio-ulna joint (DRUJ).

Building on the ABCs method of evaluation, as introduced in Chapter 1, and assuming that adequacy has been checked, **Table 4.2** outlines the specific checks related to the evaluation of radius and ulna images, such as evaluating the joints, which are often on the periphery of the image; dedicated images must be considered if they cannot be clearly seen. **Figure 4.1** demonstrates normal anteroposterior (AP) and lateral radius and ulna images, summarising these additional checks for radius and ulna images, which will be discussed in more detail in this chapter.

Table 4.2 Summary of the ABCs method of evaluation for the radius and ulna.

Focus	Points to consider
Bones	Pay particular attention to the distal radial metaphysis in children and the radial head and neck in adults.
	The ulna, and occasionally the radius, in children can be bowed in a plastic bowing fracture.
Cartilaginous areas	Check that the carpus and distal radius is normally aligned (see Chapter 3 for further guidance on assessing this).
	Check radiocapitellar alignment, if this can be seen on the images (see Chapter 5 for further guidance on assessing this).
	Check the distal radio-ulnar alignment for widening.
Soft tissues	Soft tissues around the elbow joint may demonstrate an effusion (see Chapter 5 for further guidance on assessing this).
	The pronator quadratus fat stripe must be in close contact with the distal radius (see Chapter 3 for further guidance on assessing this).

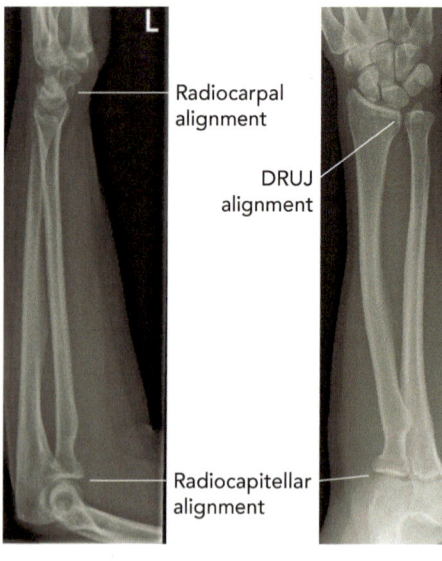

Radiocarpal alignment

DRUJ alignment

Radiocapitellar alignment

Figure 4.1 (a) AP and (b) lateral radius and ulna images demonstrating checks unique to this area.

BONES

- The radius or ulna could have a bowing appearance in a child without a visible fracture (**Figure 4.2**). An injury called a **plastic bowing fracture** can occur when a fall onto the outstretched hand (FOOSH) results in a longitudinal compression. The resultant force causes the bone to bend, with multiple micro-fractures on the concave side of the bone. This is more common in the ulna, but may be seen in both bones and can also occur with an associated fracture in the opposing bone.

- An isolated ulna fracture can be associated with a **Monteggia**-type fracture dislocation, so the elbow needs to be clearly seen in two projections (**Figure 4.3**). It can also be a **defence injury**, so correlation with clinical history is important, particularly in vulnerable patients (see Section 5 for further detail).

- Care must be taken when looking at the periphery of the image, as subtle fractures may be missed.

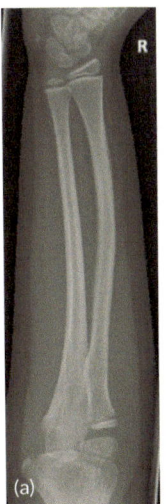 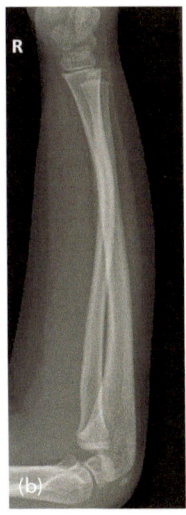

Figure 4.2 (a) AP and (b) lateral radius and ulna images demonstrating a plastic bowing fracture of the radius.

> **Comment:** bowing deformity in the midshaft of the radius indicating a plastic bowing fracture.

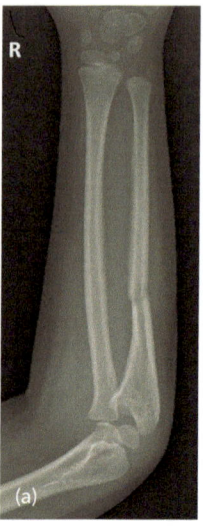
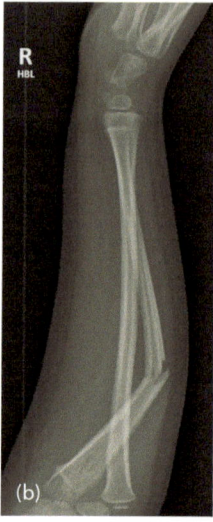

Figure 4.3 (a) Posteroanterior and (b) lateral radius and ulna images demonstrating an ulna fracture and radial head displacement; elbow projections are needed.

Comment: anteriorly angulated ulna midshaft fracture and laterally dislocated radial head.

CARTILAGINOUS AREAS

- Wrist and elbow joints should be assessed using techniques outlined (see Chapters 3 and 5, respectively). This is particularly important if there is an isolated radius or ulna fracture with no other obvious fracture present, as the ring has been breached and a second injury needs to be identified. It may be difficult to assess the wrist and elbow joints if they are at the periphery of the collimated area, and it may be necessary to obtain dedicated joint images.

- There are two injury patterns that involve disruption at the wrist or elbow joint. The **Monteggia** fracture dislocation pattern involves a fracture through the ulna midshaft and dislocation of the radiocapitellar joint, as seen in Figure 4.3. Although rare, these occur in children more often than in adults because of a FOOSH.

A **Galeazzi**-type injury, which is also caused by a FOOSH, results in a fracture of the distal third of the radius or at the junction of the distal and middle thirds, with disruption of the DRUJ (**Figure 4.4**).

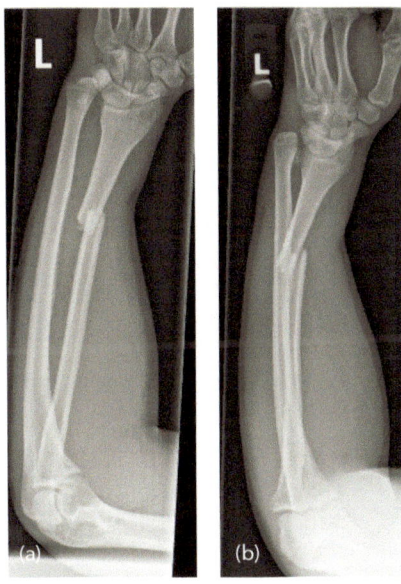

Figure 4.4 (a) Posteroanterior and (b) lateral radius and ulna images demonstrating a fracture through the radius and disruption at the DRUJ in keeping with a Galeazzi injury.

> **Comment: transverse fracture through the distal radius with posterior displacement and anterior angulation; posteromedial dislocation of the head of the ulna.**

SOFT TISSUES

- Elevation of the **pronator quadratus fat stripe** may indicate an undisplaced fracture through the distal radius or, in a child, a Salter–Harris (SH) type I injury.
- Areas of increased density may be related to retained foreign bodies, while an area of increased lucency may be due to laceration or infection. For example, a malfunctioning jet washer can cause an injury to the hands that then leads to air tracking along the fascial planes of the wrist and forearm. This may present as a small laceration, but there will be increased swelling, pain and crepitus in the soft tissues due to the air that has been injected subcutaneously under high pressure (**Figure 4.5**). This is called **subcutaneous emphysema**.

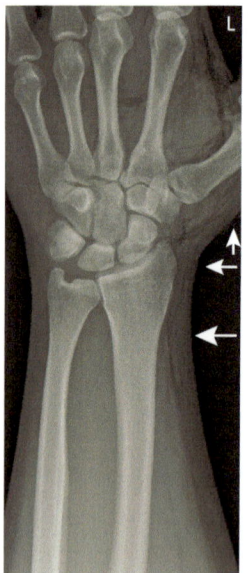 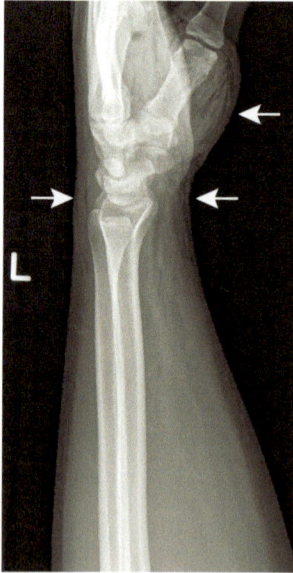

Figure 4.5 (a) Posteroanterior and (b) lateral cropped radius and ulna images demonstrating air tracking along the fascial planes of the forearm.

Comment: air within the soft tissues of the lateral wrist and forearm.

- There may be an elbow joint effusion visible on the periphery of the image, which may indicate a fracture of the radial head. This is discussed in more detail in Chapter 5.

CHAPTER SUMMARY

- Midshaft radius and ulna fractures are not usually difficult to see, as they are often displaced or angulated.
- The radius and ulna configuration is classified as a ring bone equivalent.
- The integrity of the wrist and elbow joints must be checked.
- An isolated ulna shaft fracture could cause suspicion of a defence injury in the absence of an appropriate alternative mechanism.

5. ELBOW AND HUMERUS

Injuries around the elbow joint can be subtle, and assessment of alignment and identification of fat pads is essential when searching for a possible fracture. In particular, the paediatric elbow is complex, with many ossification centres, some being fragmented. The mnemonic **CRITOE** (capitellum, radial head, internal epicondyle, trochlea, olecranon, external epicondyle) is useful, as it indicates the order of ossification, with the capitellum appearing around the age of 1 year and the others approximately every 2 years after that. Using this when evaluating paediatric elbows will help to embed normal anatomy and make identifying an abnormal appearance easier. Humeral shaft fractures occur after significant trauma and are generally displaced/angulated due to the pull of muscles. These will not be covered in detail due to the ease in identifying them; however, a spiral fracture in a young child should raise suspicion of abuse (see Chapter 13 for more detail). Proximal humerus fractures are common in older people and will be discussed in Chapter 6. Common mechanisms of injury include a direct blow and a fall onto the outstretched hand (FOOSH) and result in the injuries outlined in **Table 5.1**.

Building on the ABCs method of evaluation, as introduced in Chapter 1, and assuming that adequacy has been checked, **Table 5.2** includes the specific checks related to the evaluation of elbow images, such as evaluating the soft tissues for signs indicating possible radiologically occult fractures. **Figure 5.1** demonstrates normal anteroposterior (AP) and lateral elbow images, summarising these specific checks for elbow images, which will be discussed in more detail in this chapter.

Table 5.1 Common mechanisms of injury and associated abnormalities in the elbow.

Mechanism of injury	Typical abnormality
Direct blow	Olecranon fracture
FOOSH	Elbow dislocation with or without a coronoid fracture
	Supracondylar fracture of the distal humerus under 10 years of age
	Radial head or neck fracture above the age of 10 years
	Unicondylar fracture of the distal humerus
Throwing injury/overuse	Avulsion of the medial epicondyle

Table 5.2 Summary of systematic checks to be made when evaluating the elbow.

Focus	Points to consider
Bones	Pay close attention to the radial head and neck, as fractures here can be subtle. A Coyle's image may help if clinical symptoms indicate a fracture in this location.
Cartilaginous areas	On the lateral image, the anterior humeral line and the radiocapitellar line should pass through the mid third of the capitellum.
	In the paediatric elbow, each ossification centre must be identified and assessed, ensuring that those expected for the age of the child are present and normally located. CRITOE will help in assessing displacement of any of the ossification centres. Each visible ossification centre should be closely aligned with the adjacent bone without any widening at the growth plate, which may indicate avulsion.
Soft tissues	On the lateral image, the visibility of a posterior fat pad indicates an effusion and may be associated with trauma.
	Also on the lateral image, the supinator fat stripe should be closely associated with the proximal radius.

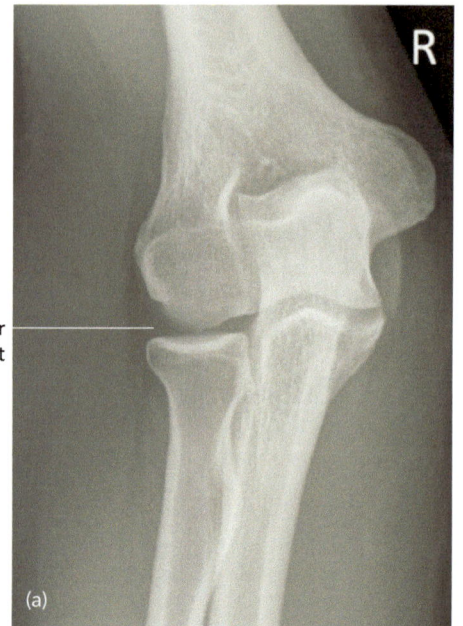

Radiocapitellar
alignment

(a)

R

Anterior
humeral
line

Posterior
fat pad
location

(b)

R

Anterior fat pad

Supinator fat stripe

Coronoid process

Radiocapitellar
alignment

Figure 5.1 (a) AP and (b) lateral elbow images demonstrating the checks that are unique to this area.

BONES

- The cortices must be assessed, paying particular attention to the **radial neck and head**. Fractures here can be very hard to see (**Figure 5.2a**). A Coyle's projection may be beneficial. Occasionally the fracture may be impacted and the only evidence of this will be a sclerotic line. There may also be an effusion, but do not be misled by the absence of one, as the radial neck lies outside the joint capsule and a fracture here does not necessarily cause an effusion.
- Fractures involving the **olecranon process** are often distracted (**Figure 5.2b**).

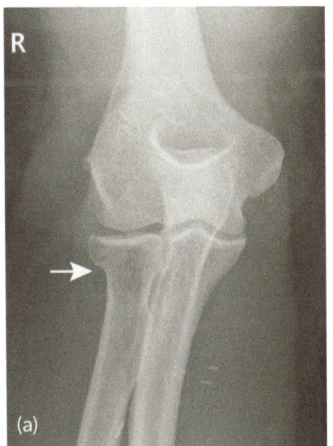 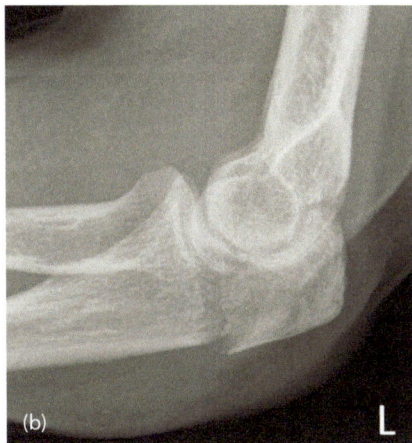

Figure 5.2 (a) AP elbow image demonstrating a radial head fracture. (b) Lateral elbow image demonstrating a distracted olecranon process fracture.

- The **coronoid process** may be fractured, and this may be evident only on the lateral elbow image (**Figure 5.3**). It is associated with elbow dislocation, or attempted dislocation, when the distal humerus moves anteriorly, impacting the coronoid process.
- The radial nerve lies in the spiral groove of the humerus, putting it at risk of damage in a displaced fracture (**Figure 5.4**). If the

nerve becomes trapped in the fracture, the patient may suffer loss of sensation in the lower arm and wrist drop. This is known as a Holstein–Lewis fracture.

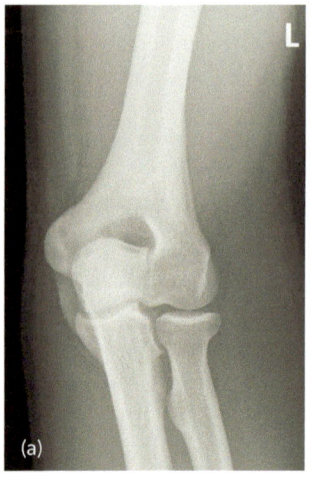
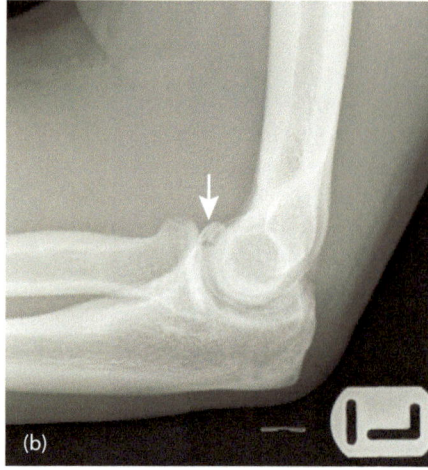

Figure 5.3 (a) AP and (b) lateral elbow images demonstrating a lucent line through the coronoid process indicating a fracture.

Comment: intra-articular coronoid process fracture with effusion.

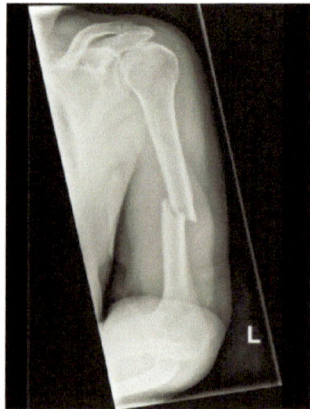

Figure 5.4 AP humerus image demonstrating a displaced fracture.

- Children under the age of 10 years tend to sustain **supracondylar fractures** with a FOOSH, with this being the most common fracture in children under the age of 7 years.[1] They can be very subtle (**Figure 5.5a**), and other signs of fracture should be assessed, such as the presence of an effusion and/or displacement of the alignment lines. Both are discussed later in this chapter. The degree of displacement or angulation can vary, with some injuries demonstrating significant deformity (**Figure 5.5b**). In these instances, the brachial artery and median nerve, which run in close contact with the anterior aspect of the distal humerus, are at risk of damage from the sharp fracture fragment stretching these structures or from entrapment in the fracture.

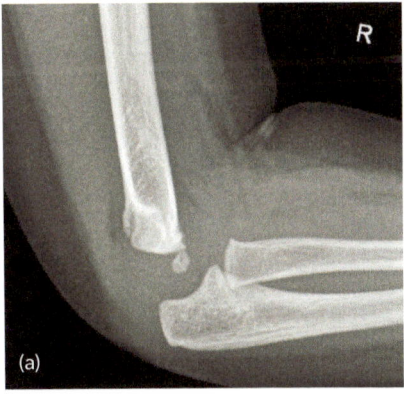 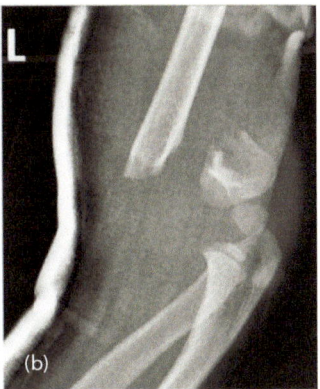

Figure 5.5 Lateral paediatric elbow images demonstrating supracondylar fractures that are (a) subtle and (b) displaced posteriorly.

- Fractures may involve a single condyle. Knowledge of CRITOE and the correct location of the ossification centres will help in differentiating between a fracture fragment and an ossification centre in a child (**Figure 5.6**). This is demonstrated in **Figure 5.7**, in which there is a bone fragment adjacent to the lateral condyle. This is unlikely to be the external epicondyle ossification centre, as the internal epicondyle and trochlea ossification centres are not yet visible.

(a)

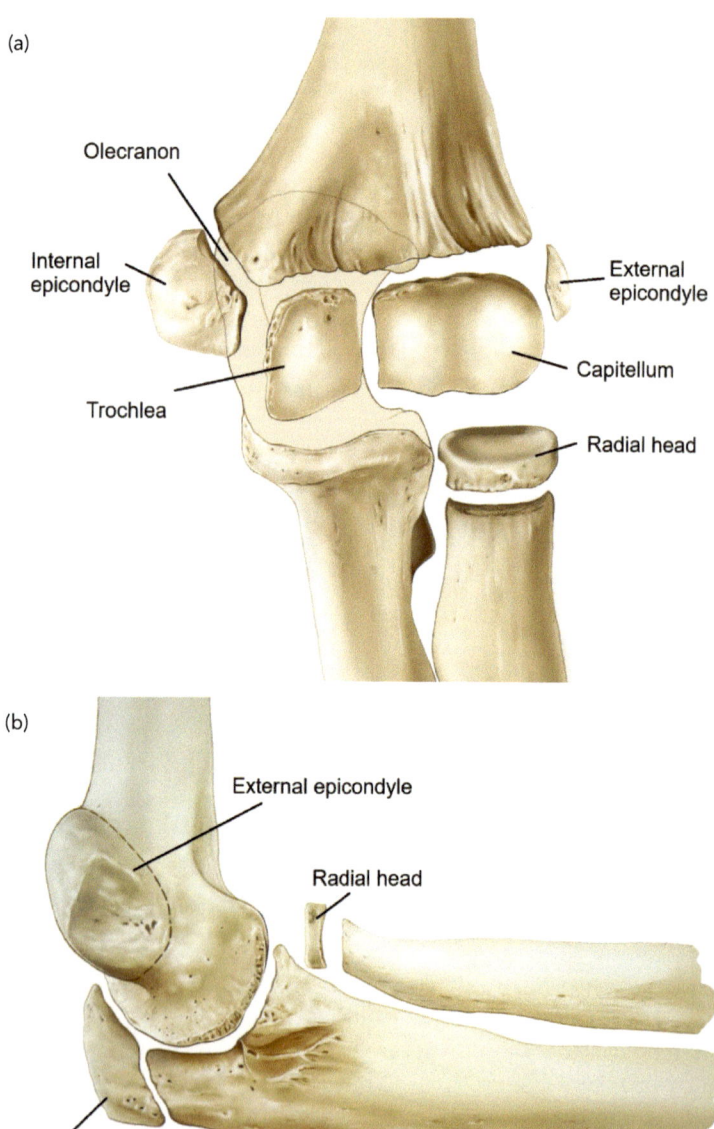

Olecranon

Internal epicondyle

External epicondyle

Capitellum

Trochlea

Radial head

(b)

External epicondyle

Radial head

Olecranon

Figure 5.6 Schematic of the location of ossification centres in the elbow demonstrated from (a) the front and (b) the side.

- Occasionally, a child may present with pain in the proximal humerus, which is excessive for the injury sustained. X-ray examination may reveal a pathological fracture through a simple bone cyst (see Section 5).

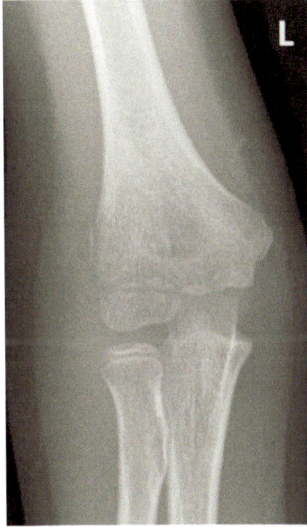

Figure 5.7 AP paediatric elbow image demonstrating a fracture of the external epicondyle.

CARTILAGINOUS AREAS

- There are many growth plates associated with the ossification centres, which can be damaged, resulting in avulsion of the ossification centre. As well as assisting in differentiating a fracture from an ossification centre, knowledge of the order of ossification will also help in identifying ossification centres that are not correctly positioned. '**Little league**' elbow is an injury that may be overlooked in children, in which the ulnar collateral ligament pulls on the internal epicondyle, resulting in its avulsion. The epicondyle may displace into the joint space, mimicking the trochlea (**Figure 5.8**). If the trochlea is seen but the internal epicondyle is not, suspicion of avulsion should be suggested. A joint effusion should not be relied on to support this type of injury, as the epicondyles lie outside the capsule and a joint effusion may not be visible.

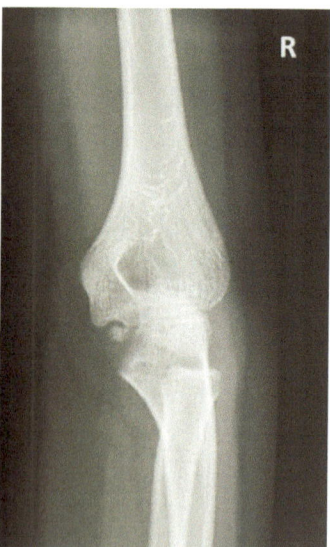

Figure 5.8 AP elbow image demonstrating an area of ossification in the position of the trochlea but without ossification of the internal epicondyle, suggesting that this is an avulsed internal epicondyle.

■ The elbow is the second most common joint to be dislocated, and it is more prevalent in adults than in children.[2] The mechanism of injury is usually a fall onto the hyperextended hand. Posterolateral dislocations occur most often,[2] and there can also be a fracture component, which makes the injury more complex (**Figure 5.9**). A radial head fracture is most associated with a dislocation. However, a fracture of the coronoid process may also occur, and it is essential to identify, as it can be pushed into the joint space on reduction of the dislocation. Post-reduction images need careful assessment for loose bodies within the joint space.

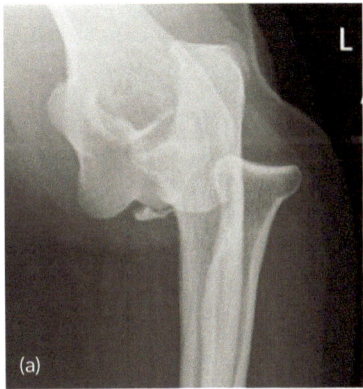 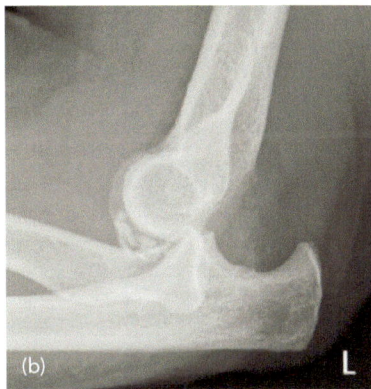

Figure 5.9 (a) AP and (b) lateral elbow images demonstrating a fracture dislocation.

> **Comment:** **posterolateral elbow dislocation with a comminuted fracture of the coronoid process.**

■ The anterior humeral line and the radiocapitellar line are useful when assessing a child's lateral elbow image.

  – The anterior humeral line should pass through the mid third of the capitellum (Figure 5.1b). If it passes through the anterior or posterior thirds, then a shift in the position of the capitellum should be considered. This can be caused by a subtle supracondylar fracture or an injury involving the distal humeral growth plate only, and may not be identified if not for a displacement such as this.

— Radiocapitellar alignment is assessed by drawing a line along the midshaft of the proximal radius, which should intersect the capitellum in the mid third (Figure 5.1b). This allows an assessment to check for displacement of the capitellum from its normal position, as well as for subluxation or dislocation at the radiocapitellar joint (**Figure 5.10**). If subluxation or dislocation of the radial head is suspected, distal radius and ulna images are needed to assess for further abnormality in this ring bone equivalent.

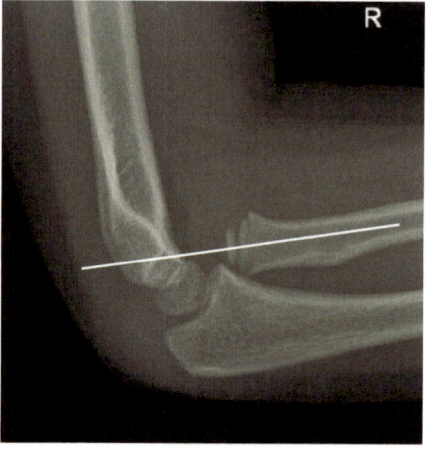

Figure 5.10 Lateral elbow image demonstrating displacement of the radiocapitellar line indicating a dislocation.

SOFT TISSUES

■ There are two fat pads closely associated with the distal humerus and within the elbow joint. When there is increased fluid within the joint because of injury, this can distend the capsule and push the fat pads away from the humerus.

- The posterior fat pad is within the olecranon fossa and cannot normally be seen on the lateral elbow image. Visualisation of the posterior fat pad indicates an effusion and has a high correlation with a bony injury. In the absence of an obvious fracture, this may indicate a radiologically occult fracture (**Figure 5.11**).
- The anterior fat pad is within the coronoid fossa on the anterior aspect of the distal humerus. It can be seen as a linear area of lucency running along the anterior aspect of the distal humerus on the lateral elbow image and separates the triceps tendon from the joint capsule. It may appear raised, referred to as 'sail like', but in the absence of a raised posterior fat pad it is unlikely to be a significant finding.

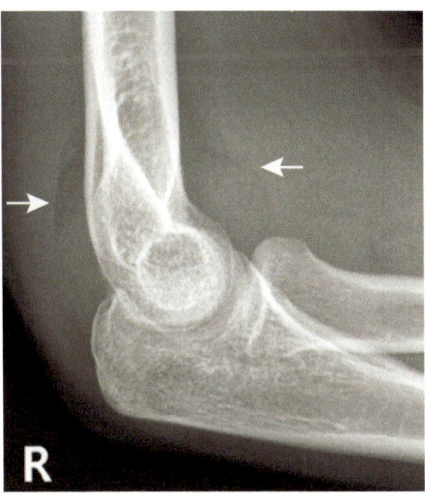

Figure 5.11 Lateral elbow image demonstrating elevation of the anterior and posterior fat pads indicating an elbow joint effusion, likely related to an occult fracture.

■ Being able to locate these on the lateral elbow image is extremely valuable in helping to identify or support the diagnosis of a subtle fracture. In a child under the age of 10 years, this may be a supracondylar fracture (Figure 5.5a) or a fracture through the distal humeral growth plate. In a child over the age of 10 years and in adult patients, this is likely to be a fracture involving the head or neck of the radius (**Figure 5.12**).

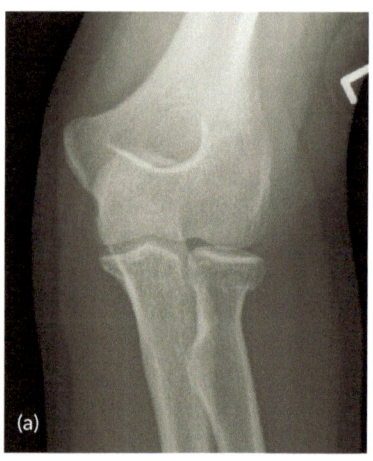 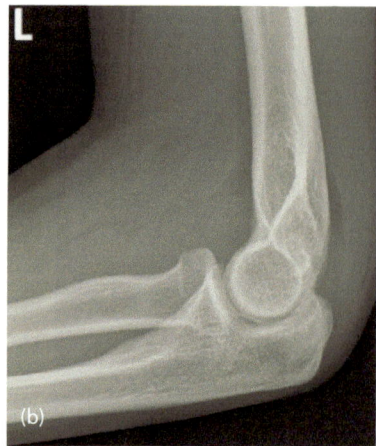

Figure 5.12 (a) AP and (b) lateral elbow images demonstrating a radial neck fracture and an effusion and raised supinator fat stripe.

> Comment: **fracture through the radial neck with an elbow joint effusion.**

- An effusion may be present in older patients with degenerative disease. If the patient has sustained trauma, care must be taken not to dismiss this effusion as degenerative in nature, and close inspection of the bones must be made to exclude a fracture.
- Do not be misled by the absence of an effusion, as the epicondyles and radial neck lie outside the joint capsule, so any injury in these areas is unlikely to cause an effusion. In addition, the fat pads may be absent if the joint capsule has ruptured, but this usually occurs only in a displaced fracture or dislocation.
- The supinator fat stripe, associated with the supinator muscle, lies along the anterior surface of the proximal radius and can be seen on the lateral elbow image (Figure 5.1b). Any bowing, elevation

or obliteration of this fat stripe may be a useful indicator of injury and is most likely to be associated with a radial neck fracture (Figure 5.12).

CHAPTER SUMMARY

- The radius and ulna should be treated as a ring bone, that is, a continuous ring and, if breached, a second injury should be sought.
- Injuries around the elbow joint can be subtle, and assessment of alignment and identification of fat pads is essential when searching for a possible fracture.
- If the posterior fat pad is seen, in the absence of an obvious fracture, this is commonly called a radiologically occult fracture, that is, there is a fracture present but it cannot be seen on the image. In adults, this fracture is generally within the radial head.

REFERENCES

1. Barr, L.V. Paediatric supracondylar humeral fractures: epidemiology, mechanisms and incidents during school holidays. *Journal of Children's Orthopaedics* 2014;8(2):167–170.
2. Robinson, P.M., Griffiths, E. and Watts, A.C. Simple elbow dislocation. *British Elbow and Shoulder Society* 2017;9(3):195–204.

6. PROXIMAL HUMERUS AND SHOULDER

The shoulder is the most mobile and unstable joint, making it prone to dislocation in adults.[1] In children, dislocations are rare, but they are at risk of a fracture involving the proximal humeral growth plate or the clavicle, with the latter being the most common of all children's fractures.[2] Fractures in adults are often associated with osteoporosis and involve the surgical neck of the humerus (between the tuberosities and the deltoid tubercle) or the anatomical neck of the humerus (proximal to the surgical neck), the latter leading to osteonecrosis. Common mechanisms of injury are high-energy trauma in the young and simple fall onto the outstretched hand (FOOSH) in older people (**Table 6.1**).

An important element of shoulder evaluation is a review of the lung fields. While this text does not cover evaluation of the chest image in detail, it is important to be able to recognise abnormalities that may need an urgent report or immediate treatment.

Building on the ABCs method of evaluation, as introduced in Chapter 1, and assuming that adequacy has been checked, **Table 6.2** includes the specific checks required for images of the shoulder and proximal humerus, including the numerous measurements, which are reliant on good radiographic technique. **Figure 6.1** demonstrates normal anteroposterior (AP) and axial shoulder images, summarising these additional checks for images of the shoulder and proximal humerus, which will be discussed in more detail in this chapter.

Table 6.1 Common mechanisms of injury and associated abnormalities in the proximal humerus and shoulder.

Mechanism of injury	Typical abnormality
Direct blow	Transverse fracture to the humerus Greater tuberosity fracture Clavicle or scapular fracture
FOOSH	Surgical or anatomical neck of the humerus fracture Transverse fracture to the humeral shaft Clavicle fracture Dislocation/subluxation of the GHJ or ACJ
High-energy trauma	Dislocation of the GHJ or ACJ Fracture of the humeral neck or clavicle
Seizure or electric shock	Posterior dislocation

ACJ, acromioclavicular joint; GHJ, glenohumeral joint.

Table 6.2 Summary of systematic checks to be made when evaluating the humerus and shoulder.

Focus	Points to consider
Bones	On a well-positioned AP shoulder image, the proximal humerus will have the appearance of a walking stick because of external rotation of the arm from the shoulder joint. Greater tuberosity fractures may be missed on a poorly positioned AP image. Osteonecrosis may occur in the humeral head following injury involving the anatomical neck. Ribs and the thoracic spine must be assessed for abnormality.
Cartilaginous areas	Check the glenohumeral, acromioclavicular and sternoclavicular joints for alignment. Normal distances are: • acromioclavicular joint, 6 mm (female); 7 mm (male); • coracoclavicular distance, 11–13 mm; • subacromial space, 7–11 mm.
Soft tissues	There should be no areas of increased density within the soft tissues, which, if present, may be related to calcific tendonitis in the rotator cuff or biceps tendons. There should be no areas of diffuse subcutaneous lucency, which may indicate traumatic emphysema as a result of pneumothorax. It is important to check the lungs for any lesion, pneumothorax or signs of infection.

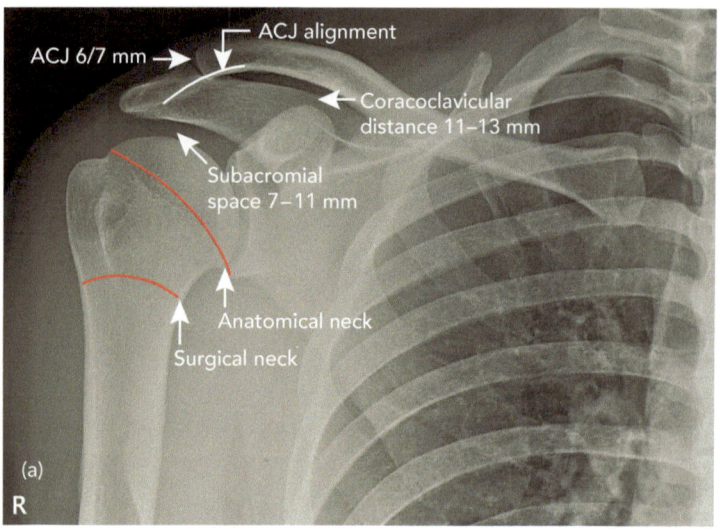

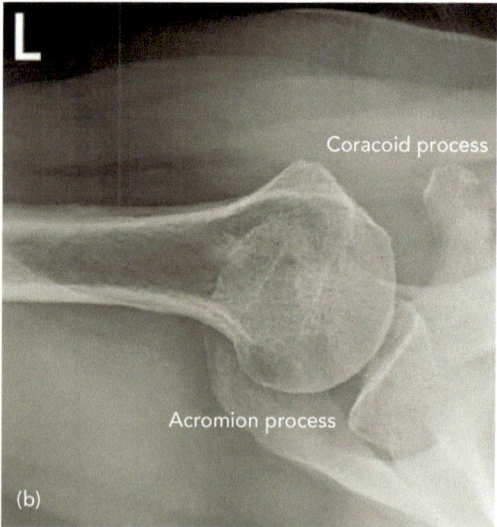

Figure 6.1 (a) AP and (b) axial shoulder images demonstrating the checks that are unique to this area. ACJ, acromioclavicular joint.

BONES

- A fracture through the **greater tuberosity**, caused by a fall onto the lateral aspect of the shoulder, is often difficult to see, and a well-positioned AP shoulder image is needed to fully appreciate it (**Figure 6.2**). Isolated greater tuberosity fractures account for almost 20% of all proximal humeral fractures.[3] More commonly, a greater tuberosity fracture is associated with a fracture through the neck of the humerus.

- A fracture of the **anatomical neck of the humerus**, caused by FOOSH, runs obliquely in the location of the closed physeal plate (**Figure 6.3a**). These fractures can result in **osteonecrosis** of the humeral head due to interruption of the blood supply, so careful evaluation of the subarticular bone is needed on the follow-up images, looking for the initial sclerosis followed by the breakdown of the bone.

- A fracture of the **surgical neck of the humerus** is more common than of the anatomical neck of the humerus and often occurs in osteoporotic patients following a FOOSH (**Figure 6.3b**). It may also involve avulsion fractures of the lesser and greater tuberosities. There may be an element of impaction at the fracture site, and the head of the humerus often angulates posteriorly.

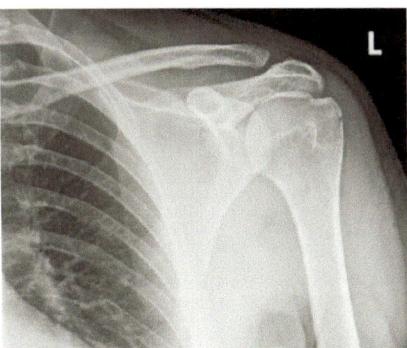

Figure 6.2 AP shoulder image demonstrating a greater tuberosity fracture.

Comment: fracture through the greater tuberosity.

- In older patients, the deltoid tuberosity can demonstrate some cortical thickening. This appearance can be seen in Figure 6.3a.

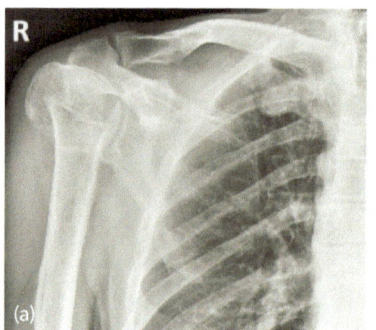
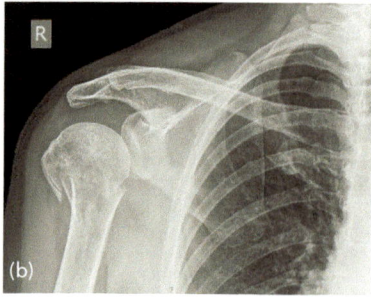

Figure 6.3 AP shoulder images demonstrating fractures through the (a) anatomical neck of the humerus and (b) surgical neck of the humerus.

- Irregularity may be seen, in the form of a depression, in the posterior aspect of the humeral head in a patient who has suffered an anterior shoulder dislocation. This is a **Hill–Sachs lesion**, caused by the impact of the head of the humerus as it attempts to relocate within the glenoid cavity (**Figure 6.4**).

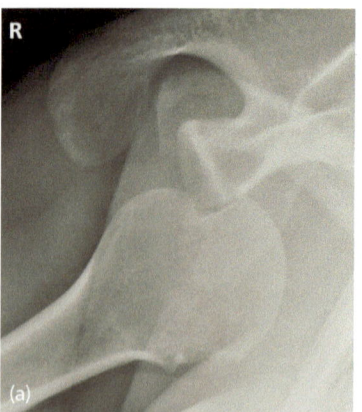
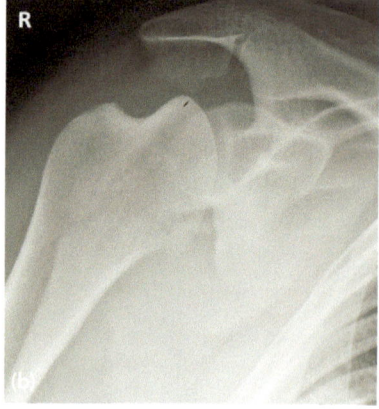

Figure 6.4 Modified axial shoulder images demonstrating (a) impaction of the head of the humerus on the glenoid in an anterior shoulder dislocation and (b) irregularity in the posterior humeral head indicating a Hill–Sachs lesion.

- Clavicle injuries, caused by a direct blow or FOOSH, need dedicated clavicle projections. Around 75% of clavicle fractures are in the middle third, with the remaining being in the distal (20%) or the proximal (5%) thirds. A single image may not enable an undisplaced fracture to be seen or demonstrate the full extent of an injury (**Figure 6.5**). However, clavicle fractures are generally associated with an angular deformity due to the pull of the sternocleidomastoid muscle, which is attached medially and pulls the fragment superiorly, and the pectoralis muscle, which pulls the lateral aspect of the clavicle inferiorly (**Figure 6.6**).

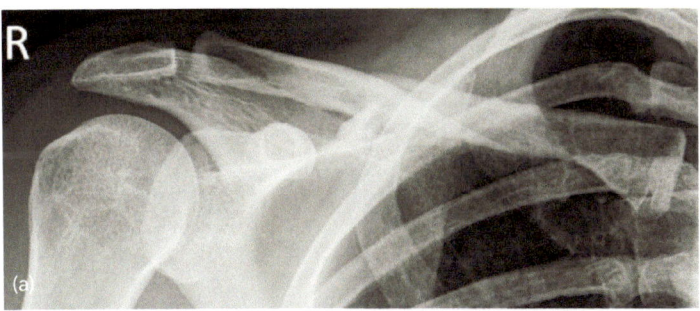

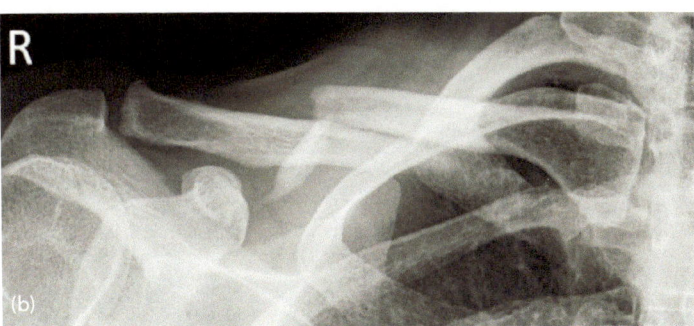

Figure 6.5 (a) AP and (b) infero-superior images of the clavicle demonstrating a fracture.

Comment: comminuted fracture through the midshaft of the clavicle with posterior displacement.

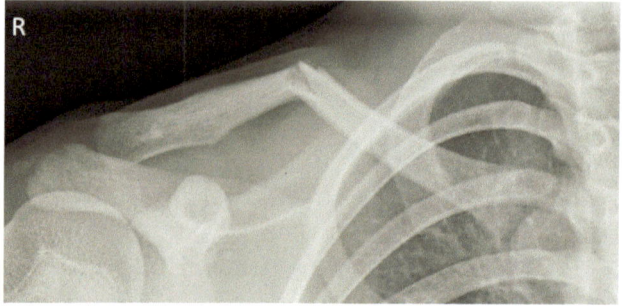

Figure 6.6 AP clavicle demonstrating an angulated midshaft fracture.

- The scapula may be difficult to see, and a dedicated lateral scapula projection is helpful if an injury in this region is suspected. There are associated injuries, such as rib fractures, in 89% of cases[4] (**Figure 6.7**). Fractures of the scapula usually result from high-energy blunt trauma either directly to the scapula or through a high-energy FOOSH; however, if a scapula fracture is seen in an older patient, consideration needs to be given to the mechanism of injury, as it can be caused by a physical assault.

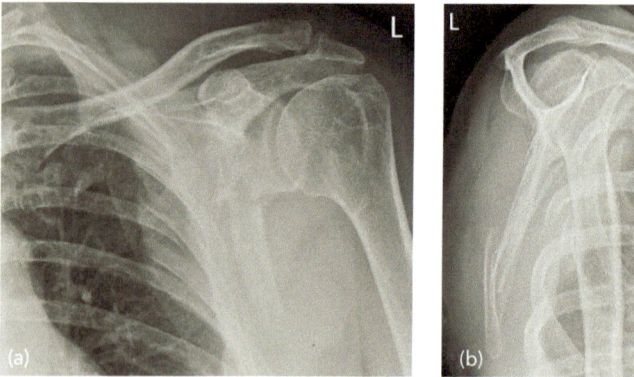

Figure 6.7 (a) AP shoulder and (b) lateral scapula images demonstrating a fracture through the scapula body and rib fractures.

> **Comment: comminuted fracture through the scapula and multiple rib fractures.**

- An important area of the scapula to assess in a patient who has dislocated their shoulder anteriorly is the inferior rim of the glenoid. A small avulsion fracture can occur here, called a **Bankart lesion**. This occurs when the humeral head impacts with the glenoid labrum resulting in a tear of the labrum, which will not be seen on the image, or a fracture through the inferior glenoid rim (**Figure 6.8**).

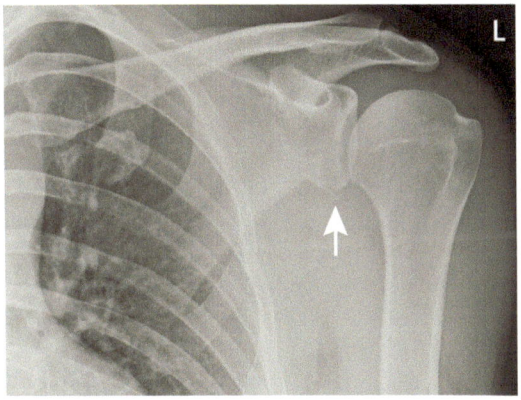

Figure 6.8 AP shoulder image demonstrating an avulsion fracture from the inferior glenoid rim.

> **Comment: there is a bony Bankart lesion at the inferior glenoid.**

- Shoulder **impingement** is a common presentation for shoulder pain. It occurs when there is damage to the rotator cuff, which passes through the subacromial space, and it can no longer hold the head of the humerus within the glenoid cavity. The head of the humerus moves superiorly, resulting in impaction with the acromion process when the arm is abducted. Other causes of impingement include developmental anomalies of the acromion process. A curved or hooked acromion process will impact the head of the humerus, leading to irregularity and increased sclerosis in this area (**Figure 6.9**).

- If a patient has sustained blunt trauma to the shoulder, there is a possibility of rib fractures (Figure 6.7). With significant trauma, a rib may be fractured in two or more places, referred to as a **flail segment** (**Figure 6.10**). This has an impact on the normal respiratory processes and can lead to a lack of aeration within a lung segment. These could be seen on shoulder images, but the patient is also likely to have a chest X-ray if they have had significant trauma. While the focus is on shoulder imaging, it is important to highlight the need to comment on fractures that are visible on a chest image. The complications associated with rib fractures, such as a pneumothorax, should also be assessed and this will be discussed later in this chapter. Follow local protocols when considering making a comment on a chest image.

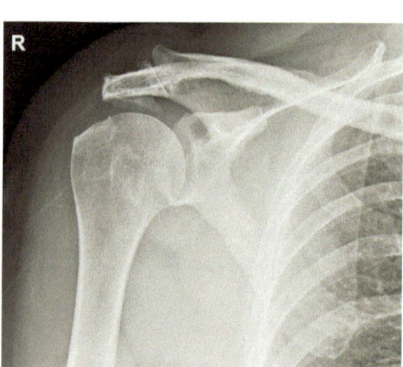

Figure 6.9 AP shoulder image demonstrating a hooked acromion process with irregularity and slight increased sclerosis at the greater tuberosity in keeping with impingement.

Comment: no fracture or dislocation; signs of impingement at the greater tuberosity.

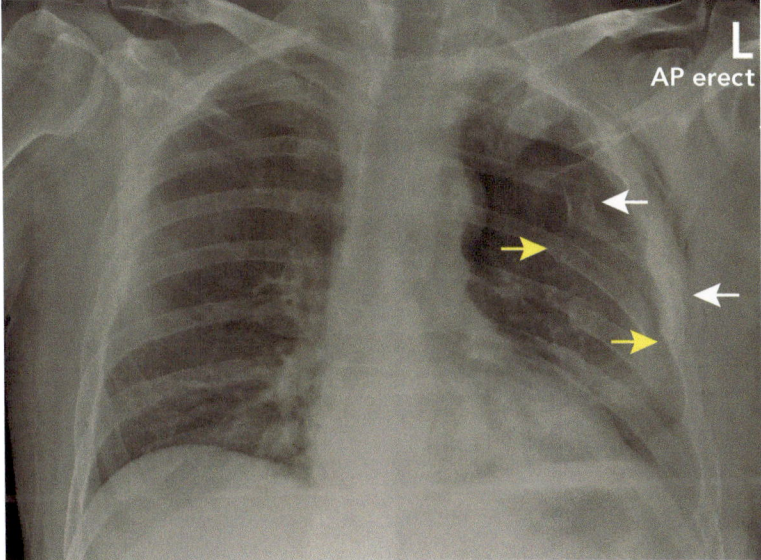

Figure 6.10 AP chest image demonstrating multiple left-sided rib fractures.

> **Comment:** **multiple left-sided rib fractures with a flail segment visible at the left fourth and fifth ribs; there is traumatic emphysema, suggesting a pneumothorax is present.**

CARTILAGINOUS AREAS

- Glenohumeral alignment is assessed by ensuring that the humeral head articulates with the glenoid cavity and the two articular surfaces are congruous. Occasionally, a subluxation will occur, which is either traumatic or caused by an **effusion** within the shoulder capsule, which forces the head of the humerus inferiorly (**Figure 6.11**).

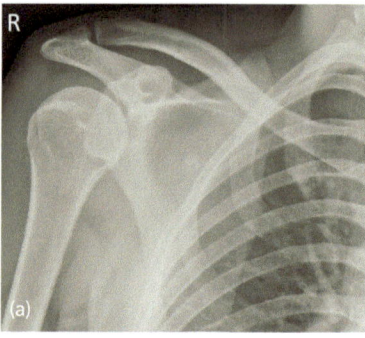
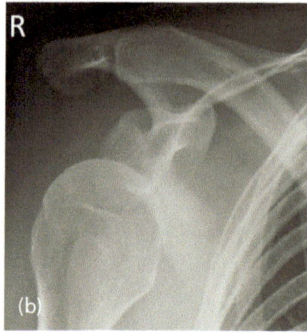

Figure 6.11 (a) AP and (b) modified axial shoulder images demonstrating inferior subluxation caused by a large effusion.

> **Comment:** inferior subluxation at the glenohumeral joint and a large effusion.

- The head of the humerus most often dislocates anteriorly. It will lose congruity with the glenoid cavity on both AP and axial images and move anteriorly and inferiorly towards the coracoid process (**Figure 6.12**).

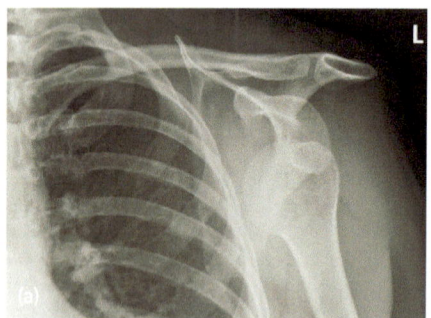
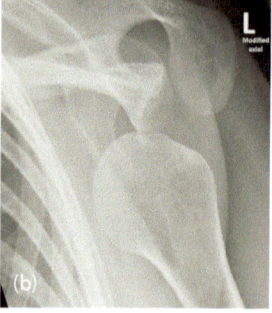

Figure 6.12 (a) AP and (b) modified axial shoulder images demonstrating anterior dislocation.

> **Comment:** anterior dislocation of the glenohumeral joint.

- The head of the humerus should look like a **walking stick** on a correctly positioned AP shoulder image (**Figure 6.13**). Lack of external rotation of the arm will cause the head of the humerus to look like a **light bulb** (**Figure 6.14a**); however, this is also a sign of a posterior dislocation (**Figure 6.14b**). Among shoulder dislocations, 10% are posterior and these are easily missed on the AP image, so the secondary image is essential, as this helps to differentiate a true dislocation from poor technique on the AP image. The mechanism of injury for posterior dislocation can be a fall, but is more commonly a seizure or, rarely, electrocution.

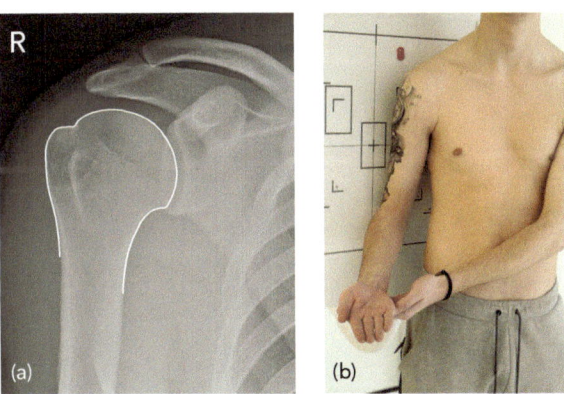

Figure 6.13 (a) Walking stick appearance of the head of the humerus. (b) Appropriate external rotation of the upper limb.

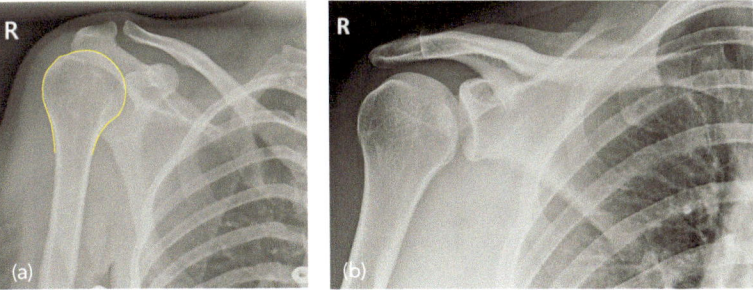

Figure 6.14 AP shoulder images demonstrating a light bulb appearance of the head of the humerus caused by (a) a lack of external rotation of the limb and (b) a posterior dislocation.

- Acromioclavicular alignment is assessed by looking at the underside of the acromion process and aligning it with the underside of the clavicle (Figure 6.1a). If the clavicle is elevated in relation to the acromion process, this will indicate a subluxation (**Figure 6.15a**) or dislocation, commonly caused by a FOOSH. With elevation of the clavicle, there may also be an increase in the coracoclavicular distance, which should measure 11–13 mm, indicating disruption of the coracoclavicular ligament (**Figure 6.15b**). The acromioclavicular joint (ACJ) can be widened without malalignment, greater than 6 mm in females and 7 mm in males. This is a simple sprain of the acromioclavicular ligament.

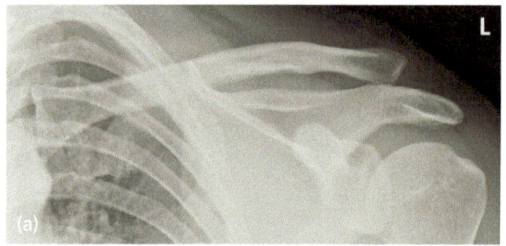

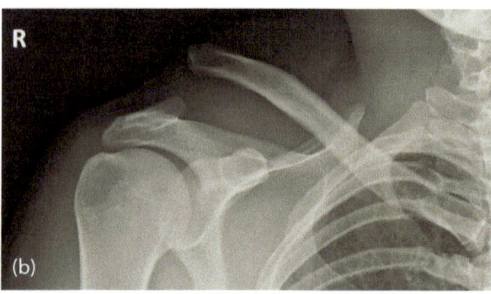

Figure 6.15 AP clavicle images demonstrating (a) subluxation of the ACJ and (b) dislocation of the ACJ with increased coracoclavicular distance.

- The sternoclavicular joint (SCJ) alignment must be assessed and oblique projections should be considered, if necessary (**Figure 6.16**). The sternal articular surface of the clavicle is larger than the opposing clavicular notch of the manubrium and only the inferior aspect of the clavicle articulates with the manubrium. SCJs rarely dislocate but, when they do, following FOOSH or direct trauma, they dislocate anteriorly or posteriorly, making it difficult to see on anterior oblique images. Posterior dislocations can cause significant trauma to the trachea, nerves and vessels, so it is essential to have focused imaging if trauma to these joints is suspected.[5] A computed tomography scan is beneficial, but a **serendipity projection** may be a quicker option to determine the integrity of the joint. This is done anteroposteriorly with a 40° cranial angle centred on the manubrium. The proximal clavicle will appear elevated in an anterior dislocation and depressed in a posterior dislocation.

- The **subacromial space** should be 7–11 mm (Figure 6.1a). Less than 7 mm indicates a **rotator cuff pathology (Figure 6.17)**. This requires a well-positioned AP shoulder image. Poor technique can have an impact on the ability to measure this space.

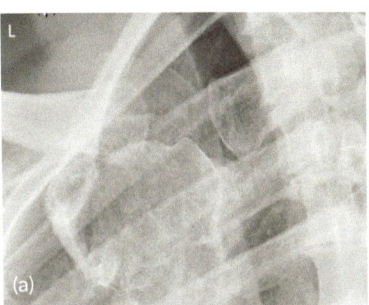 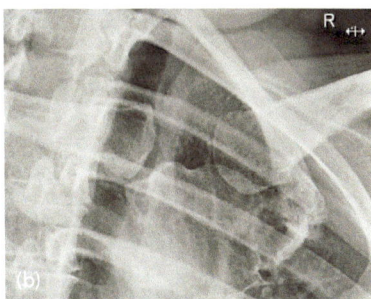

Figure 6.16 (a) Left anterior oblique and (b) right anterior oblique sternoclavicular images demonstrating normal alignment.

Comment: normal sternoclavicular joints.

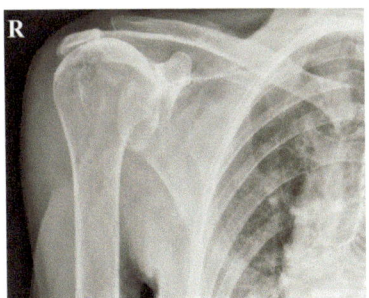

Figure 6.17 AP shoulder image demonstrating reduction in the subacromial space due to chronic rotator cuff tear.

SOFT TISSUES

- An effusion in the shoulder joint may be suspected if there is an increased density within the subacromial space and/or a **pseudosubluxation** caused by the pressure of the intra-articular fluid (Figure 6.11). A **lipohaemarthrosis** can also occur in the shoulder joint.
- Focal areas of increased density in the soft tissues may indicate calcium deposits within the rotator cuff (**Figure 6.18**). **Supraspinatus tendonitis** is most common and easily diagnosed on an AP image due to its location superior to the greater tuberosity (**Figure 6.19**). The remaining tendons are anterior or posterior, making it difficult to exclude a bone lesion on the AP image, as the density overlies the humeral head (**Figure 6.20a**). A secondary projection will help in differentiating between a bone lesion and tendonitis, as well as indicating which tendon is involved (**Figure 6.20b**).

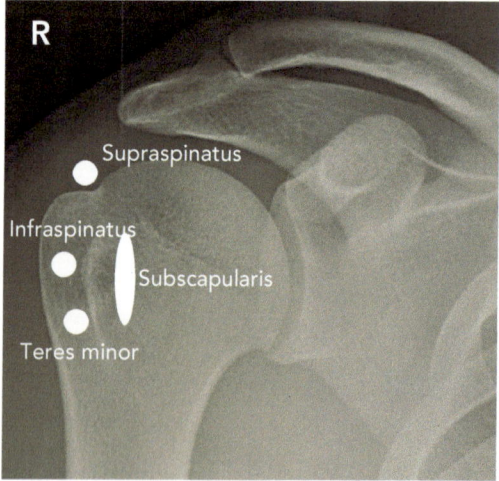

Figure 6.18 AP shoulder image with overlays demonstrating the location of deposits associated with calcific tendonitis.

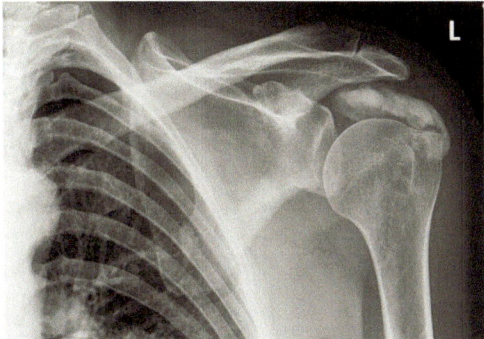

Figure 6.19 AP shoulder image demonstrating supraspinatus tendon calcification.

Comment: calcification in the soft tissues – supraspinatus tendon.

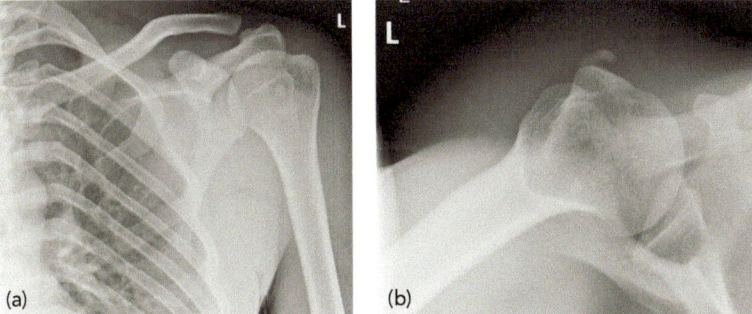

Figure 6.20 (a) AP shoulder image demonstrating a sclerotic area over the proximal humerus. (b) Axial image demonstrating that this is calcific tendonitis in the soft tissues anterior to the humerus, likely within the subscapularis tendon.

Comment: calcification in the soft tissues – subscapularis tendon.

- It is essential that the **lung fields** are evaluated. These may demonstrate known disease, which does not need any further action. A review of previous imaging will help in determining disease progression. In some cases, it will be necessary to expedite an urgent report or inform the referring clinician if immediate medical attention is needed.

- Evaluating shoulder images presents a unique opportunity to identify early signs of lung cancer. A lesion that measures more than 3 cm is referred to as a **mass** and a lesion measuring less than 3 cm is referred to as a **nodule (Figure 6.21)**. Either can be aggressive and there are typical features that help to differentiate between benign and aggressive lesions. Aggressive lesions tend to be in the upper and middle zones and have irregular margins, an absence of calcification and rapid growth when compared with previous images. It is not the role of the practitioner evaluating the images to determine if a lesion is benign or aggressive, but it is their responsibility to identify the abnormality and expedite the images for a formal report. The lesion may be a normal variant, but it is best practice to bring it to the attention of a reporting practitioner.

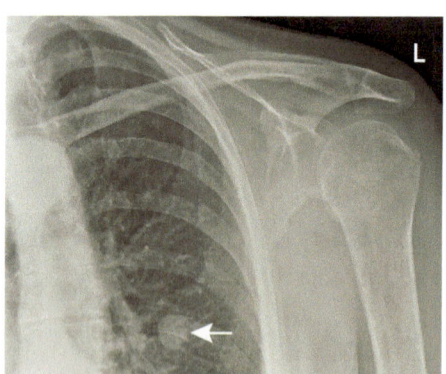

Figure 6.21 AP shoulder image demonstrating a nodule in the left lung.

Comment: lesion seen in the left lung; expedited for urgent report.

■ A **Pancoast tumour** commonly presents with shoulder pain, pain radiating down the arm or pain in the upper back, all of which are symptoms that feature on many requests for shoulder imaging.[6] This is an uncommon aggressive lesion arising in the apex of the lung (**Figure 6.22**), and any opacity seen in this region on shoulder images must be escalated for urgent report.

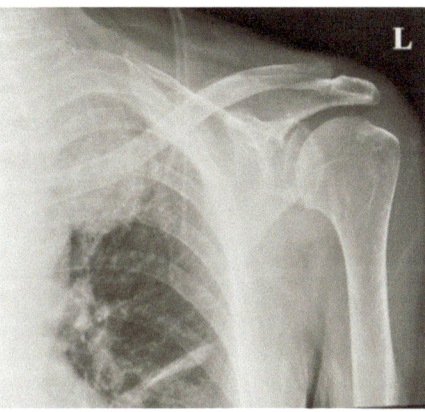

Figure 6.22 AP shoulder image demonstrating a large lesion in the left apical region indicating a Pancoast tumour.

Comment: lesion seen in the left apex; expedited for urgent report.

- The hilum should be assessed if it is visible. It is the point where the pulmonary vessels and main bronchus converge, and small lesions can be overlooked due to the complexity of this region on the image (**Figure 6.23**).

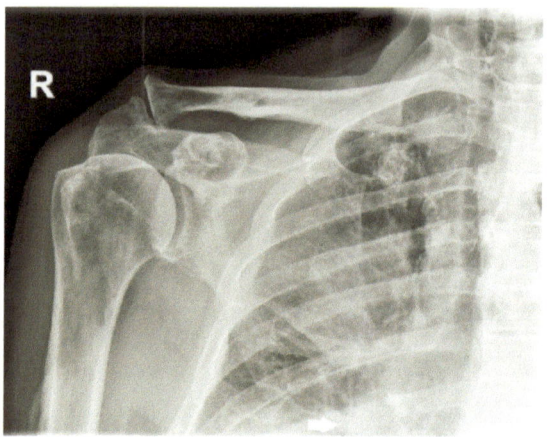

Figure 6.23 AP shoulder demonstrating a lesion hidden within the right hilum.

Comment: lesion in the right hilum; expedited for urgent report; osteoarthritis in the ACJ.

- **Lung markings** should be visible and extend to the periphery of the chest cavity where the pleural cavity is found. The pleural cavity is a space between the parietal pleura, which lines the chest wall, and the visceral pleura, which lines the lungs. This is not normally seen on an image; however, it may be visible if it contains any kind of pathology. There may be prominence of these lung markings in a patient with heart failure.
- Air leaking into the pleural cavity will separate the visceral and parietal pleura resulting in an absence of lung markings, indicating a **pneumothorax** (**Figure 6.24**). Diffuse subcutaneous emphysema may also be a sign of a pneumothorax.

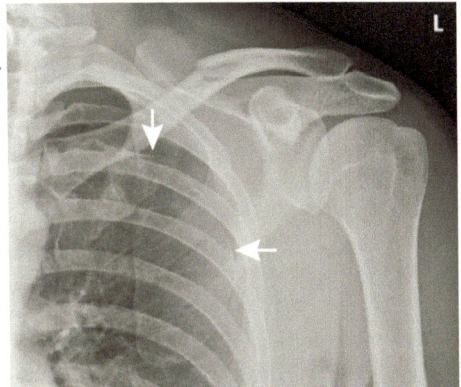

Figure 6.24 AP shoulder image demonstrating a fracture through the midshaft of the clavicle and a pneumothorax, indicated by loss of lung markings in the apical region; the lung edge can be seen.

> **Comment: fracture of the midshaft of the clavicle and pneumothorax.**

■ The pleural cavity contains a very small amount of fluid, approximately 5 ml, which acts as a lubricant for the visceral and parietal pleura. Occasionally, there may be an accumulation of fluid resulting in a **pleural effusion** being visible on the image. This is likely to be visible on the shoulder image only if either the collimation is poor and the lung base is included on the image or there is a large amount of fluid present (**Figure 6.25**). Pleural effusion can be associated with numerous conditions including infection and malignancy.

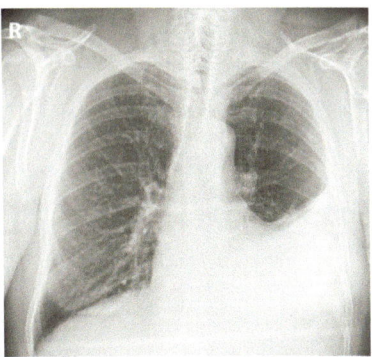

Figure 6.25 Posteroanterior chest image demonstrating a left-sided pleural effusion.

- Signs of a chest infection may be present on the image and seen as an area of patchy increased density within a single lobe, known as **consolidation (Figure 6.26)**. This is caused when the air is replaced with fluid, and there can be numerous causes, such as cancer, pneumonia or aspiration.

- A bronchus can become obstructed, by mucous, a foreign body or a tumour, and this will cause the associated lobe to **collapse** and present as an area of increased density **(Figure 6.27)**. It is often confused with consolidation, but consolidation is an area of patchy increased density, and collapse is often more even in density.

- There is a link between a chest infection and underlying lung cancer. For this reason, it is important to be able to identify infection in a timely manner so that appropriate follow-up imaging can be performed.

- Those who are qualified to interpret chest images will be able to identify the lobe affected by tumour, collapse and consolidation, but for the purposes of commenting, it is sufficient to identify that an abnormality is present and to expedite an urgent report and/or to bring the finding to the attention of the referring clinician.

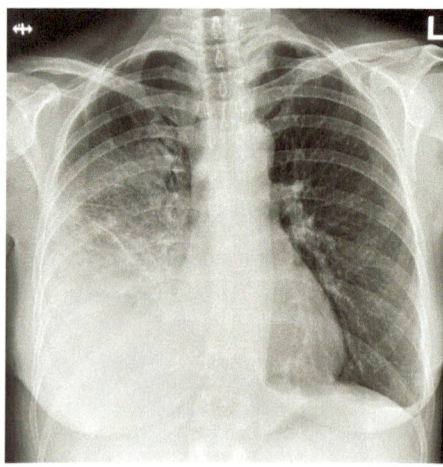

Figure 6.26 Posteroanterior chest image demonstrating right-sided consolidation.

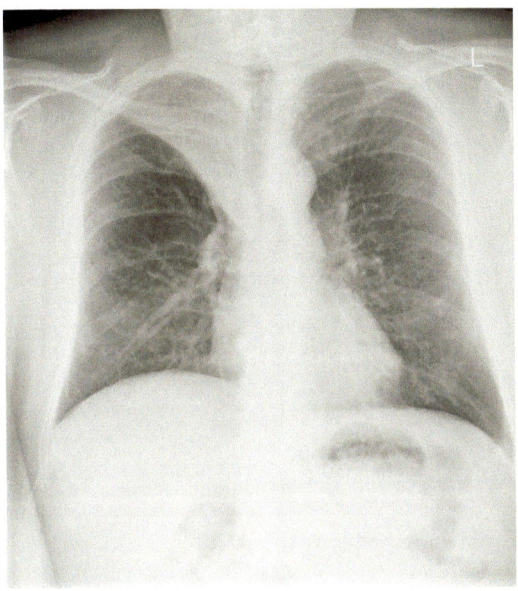

Figure 6.27 Posteroanterior chest image demonstrating a right upper lobe collapse.

- If close collimation has not been used and the diaphragm is visible on the image, it should be assessed. Referred shoulder pain can be a symptom of bowel **perforation** (see Figure 1.9).
- Occasionally, an anomaly may be seen in the right apex, which is a normal variant. The **azygos lobe** is caused by displacement of the azygos vein during embryonic development, leading to separation of a segment of the right upper lobe (**Figure 6.28**).
- Finally, if an artefact is visible on the image, it is essential to determine whether this is external or internal to the patient. All steps should be taken to determine the accurate location of the artefact (**Figure 6.29**).

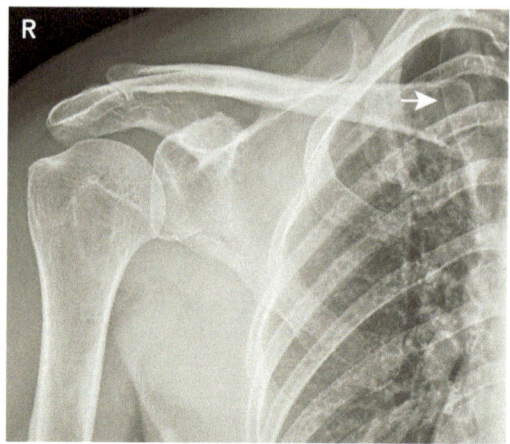

Figure 6.28 AP shoulder image demonstrating the azygos lobe.

Comment: osteoarthritis of the ACJ.

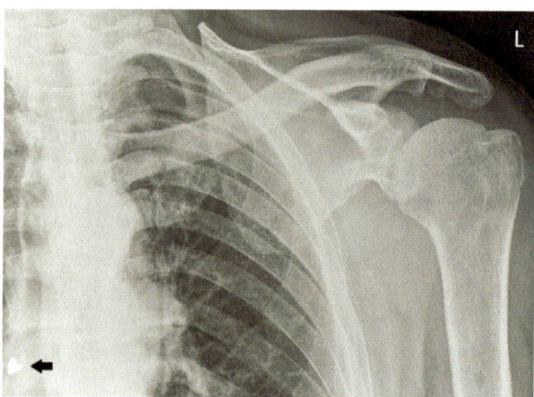

Figure 6.29 AP shoulder image demonstrating an artefact over the right hilum; investigation identified this as shrapnel internal to the patient.

Comment: fracture of the greater tuberosity; foreign body seen over the right lung, excluded as being external to the patient.

CHAPTER SUMMARY

- Looking at the whole image may result in a more clinically significant, and unexpected, finding being identified, especially in shoulder imaging where a pneumothorax or other lung pathology may be visible.
- Close attention should be paid to the lungs and any abnormal appearance expedited for urgent report.
- The humeral head articulates with the glenoid fossa and looks like a walking stick when correctly aligned. If it looks like a light bulb, this could indicate a posterior dislocation; however, a lack of external rotation of the arm can also cause this appearance.
- Glenohumeral alignment can be affected by a joint effusion and give the appearance of a subluxation.
- Reduced subacromial space could indicate a chronic rotator cuff injury.
- SCJ joints should be assessed if visible. Dedicated images may be beneficial.
- Calcification is possible within the rotator cuff.

REFERENCES

1. Shah, R., Chhaniyara, P., Wallace, W.A. and Hodgson, L. Pitchside management of acute shoulder dislocations: a conceptual review. *BMJ Open Sports and Exercise Medicine* 2017;**2**:e000116.
2. Stepanyan, H., Hennrikus, W., Flynn, D. and Gendelberg, D. Complex clavicle fractures in children: kids are not little adults. *Trauma* 2017;**21**(1):35–39.
3. Longo, U., Corbett, S. and Ahrens, P.M. Missed fractures of the greater tuberosity. *BMC Musculoskeletal Disorders* 2018;**19**:313.
4. Al-Sadek, T.A., Niklev, D., Al-Sadek, A. and Al-Sadek, L. Scapular fractures in blunt chest trauma – self-experience study. *Open Access Macedonian Journal of Medical Sciences* 2016;**4**(4):688–691.
5. Shyamasunder, B.N. and Simanchal, P.M. Sternoclavicular dislocation with fractures of the first and second ribs. *Journal of Karnataka Orthopaedic Association* 2017;**5**(1):66–68.
6. Ronan, L. and D'Souza, S. Pancoast's tumour presenting as shoulder pain in an orthopaedic clinic. *British Medical Journal Case Reports* 2013;**2013**:bcr-2012-008131.

SECTION 3
LOWER LIMB TRAUMA

7. FOOT

There are 26 bones to evaluate in the foot. In young children, the tarsus will not be fully developed. The order of ossification is as follows: calcaneum and cuboid (*in utero*), lateral cuneiform (1 year), medial cuneiform (3 years), intermediate cuneiform (4 years) and navicular (4 years). There are numerous accessory ossicles and sesamoid bones, with the addition of a number of normal variants in the child's foot.

Trauma to the foot is common, with inversion/eversion injuries occurring at any age, high-impact injuries such as in road traffic collisions or sporting injuries in young adults and stress fractures in older adults due to reduced bone density. Common mechanisms of injury and associated abnormalities are found in **Table 7.1**.

Building on the ABCs method of evaluation, as introduced in Chapter 1, and assuming that adequacy has been checked, **Table 7.2** includes the more specific checks related to the evaluation of foot images, such as assessment of midfoot alignment. **Figure 7.1** demonstrates normal dorsi-plantar (DP) and oblique foot images, summarising these additional checks for foot images, which will be discussed in more detail in this chapter.

Table 7.1 Common mechanisms of injury and associated abnormalities in the foot.

Mechanism	Typical abnormality
Crush injury	Comminuted fracture to the distal phalanx Transverse fracture through the phalanges or MTs
Stubbed toe	Fracture through the phalanges SHII fracture through the phalangeal metaphysis
Plantar- and dorsi-flexion injuries	Fracture through the bases of the phalanges, typically the proximal phalanges SHII fracture through the phalangeal metaphysis Fracture of the talus Chopart dislocation Lisfranc fracture dislocation
Inversion injury	Fracture to the base of the fifth MT Fracture of the anterior process of the calcaneum

MT, metatarsal; SHII, Salter–Harris type II.

Table 7.2 Summary of systematic checks to be made when evaluating the foot.

Focus	Points to consider
Bones	Tarsal bones should be identified by name, so as not to mistake a fractured tarsal bone for two individual bones. Always bear in mind that the lateral cuneiform is best seen on the DP oblique image and the intermediate cuneiform is best seen on the DP image. The anterior calcaneal process can be seen on a well-positioned DP oblique foot image. All visible anatomy should be assessed, including the distal tibia and fibula. It is not unusual to see malleoli fractures on foot images.
Cartilaginous areas	Calcaneocuboid and talonavicular alignment are important in assessing hindfoot/midfoot integrity. The TMTJs should be clearly seen in a well-positioned foot. Midfoot integrity is assessed by checking alignment at the second TMTJ on the DP image and the third TMTJ on the oblique image.
Soft tissues	Soft tissues should be assessed for foreign bodies obtained while walking in bare feet.

TMTJ, tarsometatarsal joint.

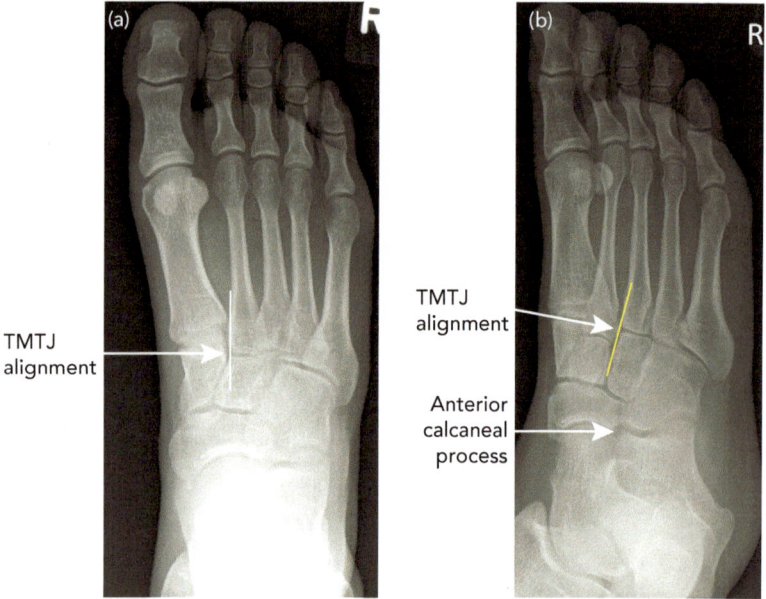

Figure 7.1 (a) DP and (b) DP oblique foot images demonstrating the checks that are unique to this area. TMTJ, tarsometatarsal joint.

BONES

- Identify the tarsal bones by name so as not to mistake a fractured tarsal bone for two individual bones. Always bear in mind that the lateral cuneiform can be clearly seen only on the DP oblique image and the intermediate cuneiform can be clearly seen only on the DP image.

- A **stress fracture** may occur in those who spend a lot of time on their feet, and it is most common in the second metatarsal (MT). The injury may not be visible at the onset of pain, and it is identifiable only once a periosteal or endosteal reaction occurs or there is callus formation (**Figure 7.2**).
- An **inversion injury** can result in a fracture to the fifth MT base. This is usually transverse and through the tuberosity commonly extending to the articular surface (**Figure 7.3a**). A fracture around 1.5 cm distal to the tuberosity, through the junction of the shaft and base of the fifth MT, may result in non-union due to disruption of the blood supply (called a **Jones fracture** (**Figure 7.3b**)).
- A common mistake in the evaluation of images of the child's foot is in the interpretation of the normal apophysis at the base of the fifth MT. The apophysis runs longitudinally whereas a fracture is often transverse (**Figure 7.4**).

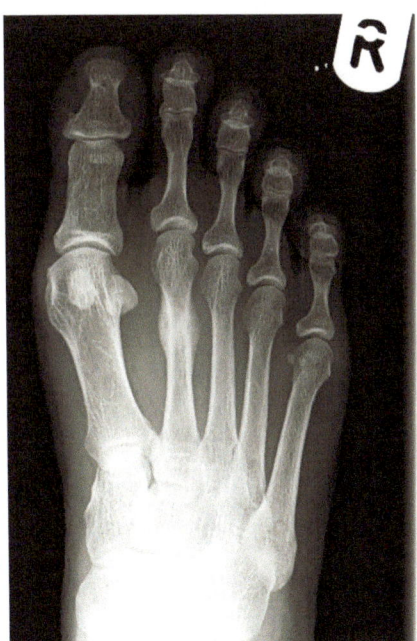

Figure 7.2 DP foot image demonstrating obvious callus formation at the midshaft of the second MT.

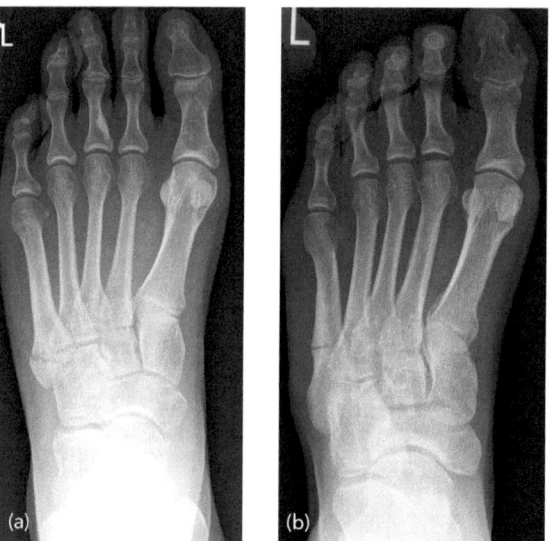

Figure 7.3 DP foot images demonstrating (a) a fracture through the tuberosity of the fifth MT and (b) a Jones fracture.

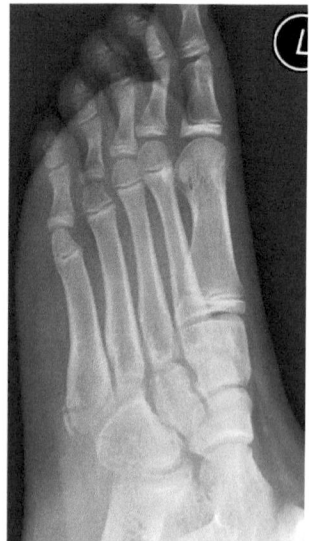

Figure 7.4 DP oblique foot image demonstrating the normal fifth MT apophysis running longitudinally adjacent to a transverse fracture through the base of the fifth MT.

- An inversion injury can result in an **anterior calcaneal process fracture**, which is visible only on a well-positioned DP oblique image (**Figure 7.5**). This is caused by excessive force being applied to the bifurcate ligament, which attaches the calcaneum to the navicular and cuboid.

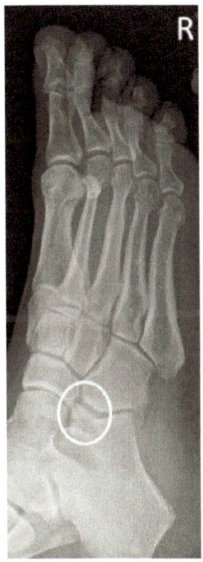

Figure 7.5 DP oblique foot image demonstrating an avulsion fracture involving the anterior process of the calcaneum.

- The lateral malleolus can be fractured in an **inversion injury**, so it must be checked on the image if visible. This is especially important in a child who may be difficult to examine and may not be able to describe the injury or verbalise the location of the pain.
- Children may present with an atraumatic limp. If there is pain and swelling in the midfoot, this may be related to **Kohler's disease**, that is, osteonecrosis of the navicular caused by a vascular disturbance to the bone (**Figure 7.6a**). The navicular will be sclerotic and possibly fragmented. However, this appearance can also be a normal variant (**Figure 7.6b**) and clinical history is key in making this diagnosis.
- Occasionally, an adolescent may present with restricted internal rotation and pain in the anterolateral aspect of the hindfoot caused by **tarsal coalition**, which occurs when two tarsal bones fuse in

either a non-osseous (cartilaginous or fibrous) or osseous (bony) coalition. The most common fusions are between the calcaneum and the navicular or talus. If the fusion is cartilaginous, there will be irregularity in the opposing margins of the two bones involved (**Figure 7.7**).

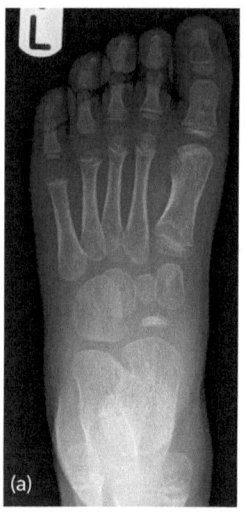

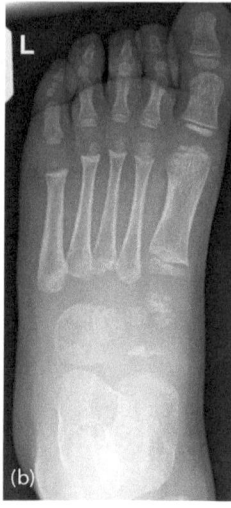

Figure 7.6 DP foot images demonstrating (a) Kohler's disease in a child with an atraumatic limp and (b) a normal variant in a child presenting after an inversion injury – note fragmentation in the medial cuneiform also.

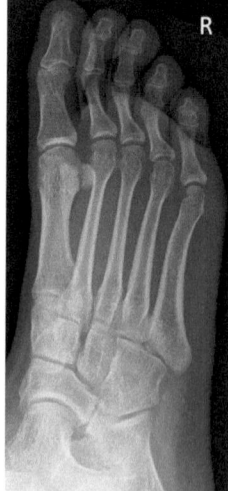

Figure 7.7 DP oblique foot image demonstrating a calcaneonavicular tarsal coalition.

CARTILAGINOUS AREAS

- The joint spaces at the tarsometatarsal joints (TMTJs), also called the Lisfranc joint complex, should be clearly seen on foot images. Integrity is evaluated by checking alignment of the medial border of the second MT with the medial border of the intermediate cuneiform on the DP image, and the medial border of the third MT with the medial border of the lateral cuneiform on the DP oblique image (Figure 7.1). Malalignment indicates disruption of the **Lisfranc ligament**, which joins the second MT base to the medial cuneiform, resulting in lateral displacement of the forefoot. A fracture may also be present, usually through the second MT base. This injury can be subtle, such as in an isolated Lisfranc injury, which is missed on 20% of images, most likely due to poor technique when there is not a 15° cranial angulation of the central ray in relation to the foot, achieved by angling the X-ray tube or elevating the toes. There is slight widening at the base of the first and second MTs (**Figure 7.8**), and there may be a 'fleck sign', that is, a small fragment of bone lying in this space.
- The less subtle injuries often involve gross lateral displacement of the second to fifth MTs, with or without lateral shift of the first MT (**homolateral injury**) (**Figure 7.9**), or lateral displacement of the second to fifth MTs and medial displacement of the first MT (**divergent injury**) (**Figure 7.10**).

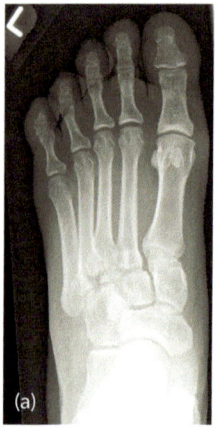 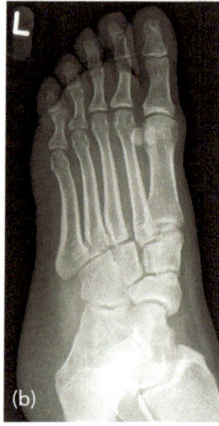

Figure 7.8 (a) DP and (b) DP oblique foot images demonstrating an isolated Lisfranc injury with a fracture of the third MT base.

Comment: fracture of the third MT base and subtle Lisfranc injury.

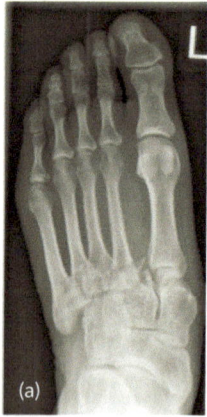 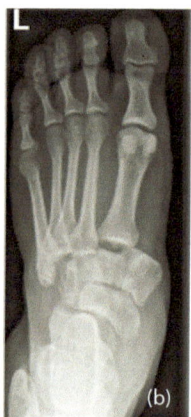

Figure 7.9 DP foot images demonstrating homolateral Lisfranc injuries with (a) lateral displacement of the second to fifth MTs and (b) lateral displacement of all metatarsals.

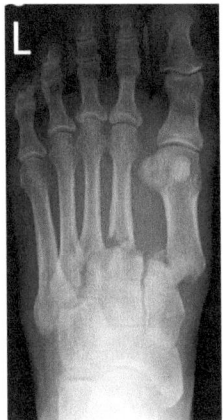

Figure 7.10 DP foot image demonstrating a divergent Lisfranc injury.

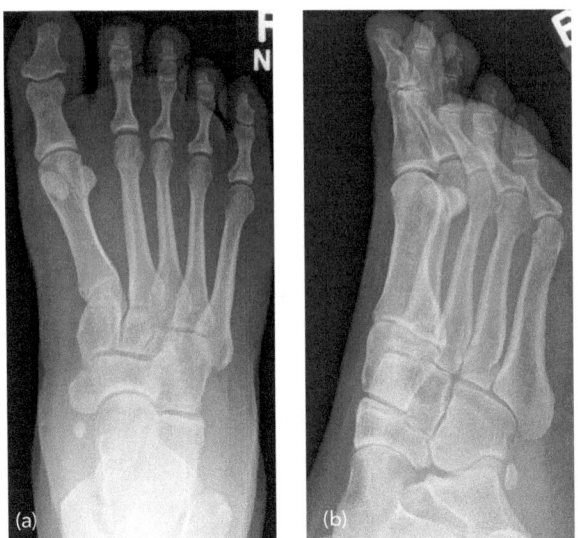

Figure 7.11 Foot images demonstrating accessory ossicles: (a) os tibiale externum and (b) os peroneum.

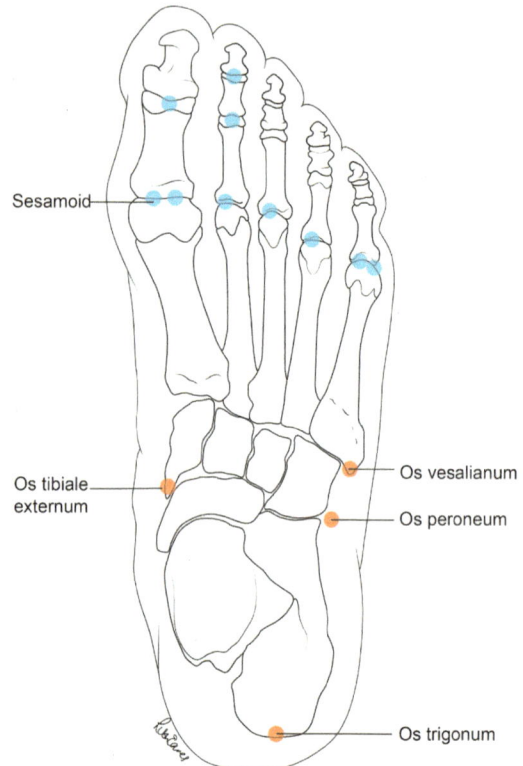

Sesamoid

Os tibiale externum

Os vesalianum

Os peroneum

Os trigonum

Figure 7.12 Location of accessory ossicles (orange) and sesamoid bones (blue) in the foot.

SOFT TISSUES

- A suspected foreign body is a common presentation in foot imaging, so soft tissues should be carefully assessed, being mindful that the visibility of a retained foreign body is dependent on its radiodensity.
- There are numerous **accessory ossicles** visible within the soft tissues around the foot (**Figure 7.11**), which can be mistaken for fractures. These lie in typical positions within the soft tissues and are rounded and corticated, so they should not be mistaken for a fracture fragment (**Figure 7.12**).

CHAPTER SUMMARY

- Some of the most subtle injuries are around the TMTJs and the anterior calcaneal process. These will be missed on poorly positioned foot images.
- Subtle changes in alignment within the TMTJs may be associated with Lisfranc fracture dislocations.
- There are many accessory ossicles around the foot and ankle, which may be misinterpreted as avulsion fractures unless the viewer familiarises themselves with the typical positions and classical appearances of these.
- The most common mistake in lower limb interpretation of children's images is related to the apophysis at the base of the fifth MT. This is a normal appearance in the growing foot, but it is easily mistaken for a fracture by the inexperienced eye.

8. ANKLE, TIBIA AND FIBULA

Adult tibia and fibula diaphyseal fractures, caused by direct trauma, twisting or compression injuries, are easy to see, but injuries specific to children, such as the **plastic bowing fracture** and the **toddler's fracture** may be a little harder to identify. The latter two injuries will be discussed in this chapter, but the main focus of the chapter is on evaluating ankle images.

The ankle is a sturdy joint created by the talus, tibia and fibula and stabilised by strong ligaments. Injuries are often caused by ankle inversion, and these range from a ligamentous sprain to trimalleolar fractures. As it is part of a 'ring bone equivalent', possible secondary injuries should be considered. Abnormalities associated with common mechanisms of injury are found in **Table 8.1**.

Building on the ABCs method of evaluation, as introduced in Chapter 1, and assuming that adequacy has been checked, **Table 8.2** includes the more specific checks related to the evaluation of ankle images, such as checking the ankle mortise to assess for stability. **Figure 8.1** demonstrates normal anteroposterior (AP) and lateral ankle images, summarising these additional checks for ankle images, which will be discussed in more detail in this chapter.

Table 8.1 Common mechanisms of injury and associated abnormalities in the ankle, tibia and fibula.

Mechanism	Typical abnormality
Inversion injury	Fracture or avulsion of the lateral malleolus Mortise disruption identified by a tilting talus Anterior calcaneal process fracture
Eversion injury	Fracture of the medial malleolus Mortise disruption
Plantar-flexion injury	Osteochondral fracture of the talar dome Talus fracture
Dorsi-flexion injury	Osteochondral fracture of the talar dome
Twisting injury	Spiral fracture
Jump from height	Fracture of the calcaneum (associated with pelvic and spine fractures)
Direct blow to lower leg	Fracture of the tibia and/or fibula
Longitudinal stress	Plastic bowing fracture

Table 8.2 Summary of the systematic checks to be made when evaluating the ankle.

Focus	Points to consider
Bones	Pay particular attention to the talar dome, assessing for an osteochondral fracture or lesion. The hindfoot, especially the fifth metatarsal base, should be assessed if it is included on the image. Gissane's and Bohler's angles can be assessed to determine calcaneal integrity. Check the anterior calcaneal process. There may be a bowing deformity of the tibia and/or fibula on the image of a child.
Cartilaginous areas	The distal fibula epiphysis should be normally aligned with the metaphysis on the AP ankle image of a child. The distal tibiofibular syndesmosis should be less than 5 mm in a skeletally mature patient. The tibiotalar joint space should be equal medially and laterally, with no greater than 2 mm difference in a skeletally mature patient, and the talar dome and tibial plafond should be parallel.
Soft tissues	Kager's triangle indicates integrity of the Achilles tendon. An ankle effusion may be seen on the lateral image anterior to the tibiotalar junction.

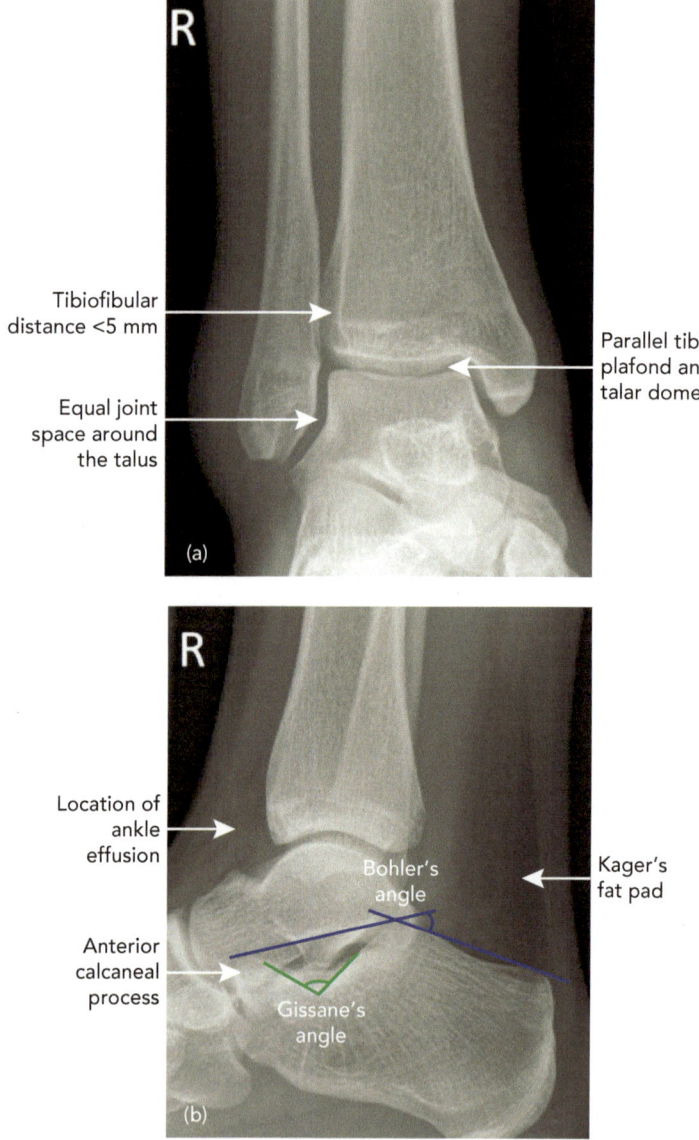

Tibiofibular distance <5 mm

Parallel tibial plafond and talar dome

Equal joint space around the talus

(a)

Location of ankle effusion

Bohler's angle

Kager's fat pad

Anterior calcaneal process

Gissane's angle

(b)

Figure 8.1 (a) AP and (b) lateral ankle images demonstrating the checks that are unique to this area.

BONES

- A **toddler's fracture** is a tibial shaft fracture in a child between 1 and 3 years of age. It can be very subtle on initial presentation and appear as a very fine linear lucency running obliquely within the tibial shaft (**Figure 8.2a**). Occasionally, there may be no abnormality seen on the initial images; however, follow-up images obtained around 7 to 10 days later will demonstrate changes consistent with an undisplaced fracture (**Figure 8.2b**). This is a common accidental injury in toddlers and not to be confused with a spiral fracture caused by physical abuse.

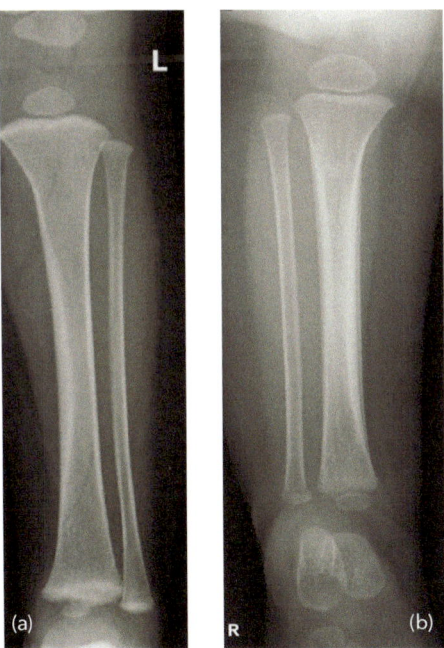

Figure 8.2 AP tibia and fibula images demonstrating (a) a lucent line in the distal tibia and (b) a tibial periosteal reaction taken on a patient whose images were normal 2 weeks earlier.

- The long bones in the lower leg of a child can undergo a subtle bending deformity resulting in a **plastic bowing fracture**. The mechanism of injury is axial loading, such as a jump from a height or impact to the foot when reaching the bottom of a slide with legs locked in extension. The bone bends when the force applied does not exceed the point at which it would break. This causes multiple micro-fractures on the concave side of the bone. The fibula is more commonly affected and is generally seen as an isolated injury (**Figure 8.3a**); however, plastic bowing fractures can also be seen in the tibia (**Figure 8.3b**). It may be overlooked, as there is no definite fracture to see, but knowledge of normal anatomy should help in identifying this injury.

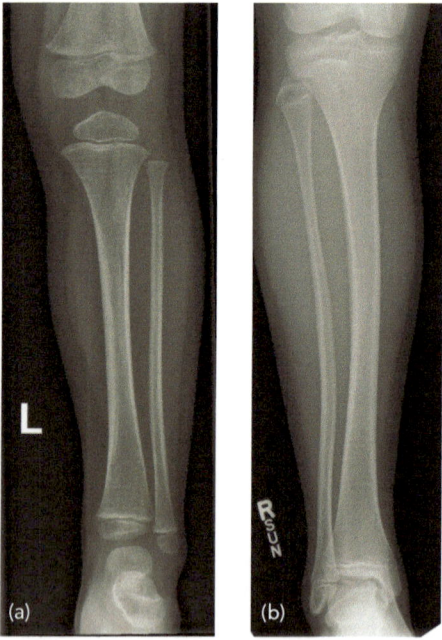

Figure 8.3 AP tibia and fibula images demonstrating (a) a plastic bowing fracture of the fibula and (b) plastic bowing fractures of both the tibia and the fibula.

- Tibial shaft fractures can fail to heal, and it is important to identify signs suggestive of delayed union in which a callus is forming but not at the normal rate or of non-union in which fracture healing has not occurred in the expected time frame.
- Medial, lateral and posterior malleoli can be fractured in an ankle injury either singularly or in any combination. The common mechanism of injury is excessive internal rotation combined with an inversion or eversion force.
- Fractures of the lateral malleolus are caused by an inversion injury. Fractures at the tip of the lateral malleolus can be subtle and can also be mistaken for an accessory ossicle. A fracture will have sharp margins, irregularity of the fragment and possible overlying soft tissue swelling. There may also be a donor site visible from which the bone fragment has been avulsed.
- Fractures through the distal fibula are classified using the **Danis–Weber classification** and are commonly referred to as Weber fractures. This classification describes the fracture position in relation to the distal tibiofibular syndesmosis.[1]

    - A **Weber A** injury is a transverse fracture through the distal fibula that is below the level of the talar dome and therefore below the level of the distal tibiofibular syndesmosis (**Figure 8.4a**).
    - A **Weber B** injury is a fracture through the distal fibula at the level of the talar dome (**Figure 8.4b**). The fracture may extend proximally, and the distal tibiofibular syndesmosis may be widened. The medial tibiotalar joint space may also be widened, suggesting deltoid ligament disruption.
    - A **Weber C** injury is a fracture through the distal fibula proximal to the distal tibiofibular syndesmosis and is often associated with a medial malleolus fracture (**Figure 8.4c**). The syndesmosis is disrupted and the medial tibiotalar joint space is often widened, suggesting a deltoid ligament injury.

Weber B and C injuries do not indicate a breach in the 'ring bone', as the injury involves disruption of the distal tibiofibular syndesmosis and a fracture of the distal fibula, so further imaging is not necessarily needed.

- A **bimalleolar fracture** involves two malleoli, usually the lateral and medial malleoli (**Figure 8.5**), and a **trimalleolar fracture** involves all three malleoli (**Figure 8.6**). It is essential that all components are identified, and 'satisfaction of search' does not result in one of these abnormalities being missed. The one most missed is the posterior malleolus fracture, as it can be obscured by the overlap of the tibia and fibula posteriorly (**Figure 8.7**).
- Pay particular attention to the talus, as, although rare, talar neck fractures are associated with trimalleolar fractures.

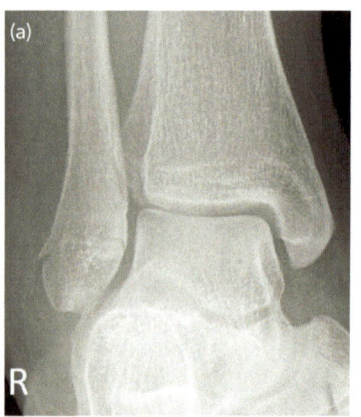
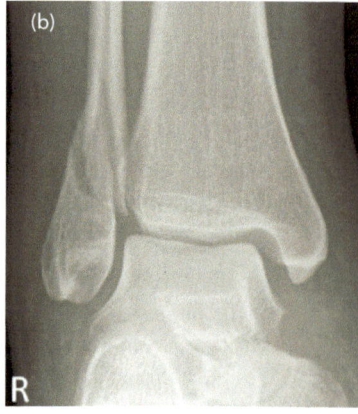
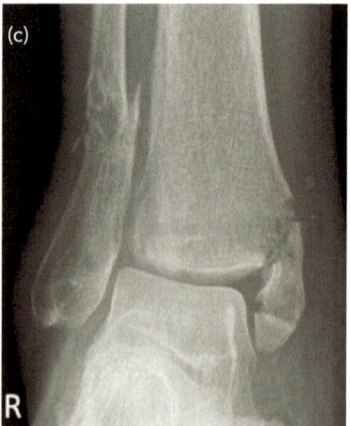

Figure 8.4 AP ankle images demonstrating (a) a Weber A fracture, (b) a Weber B fracture and (c) a Weber C fracture.

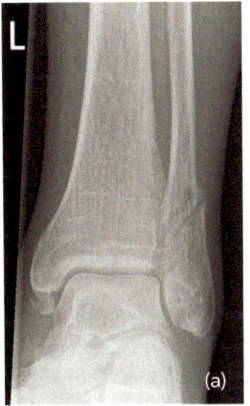
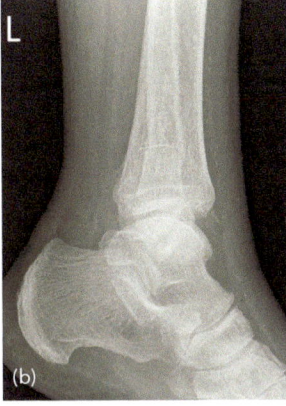

Figure 8.5 (a) AP and (b) lateral ankle images demonstrating a bimalleolar fracture.

Comment: oblique distal fibula fracture and transverse intra-articular medial malleolus fracture; normal alignment at the mortise: Weber type B.

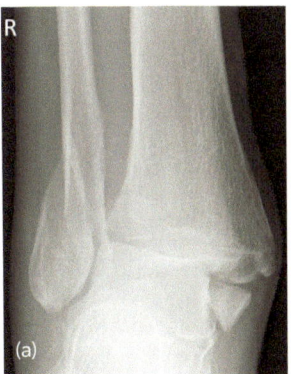
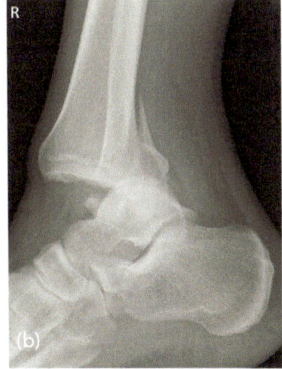

Figure 8.6 (a) AP and (b) lateral ankle images demonstrating a trimalleolar fracture dislocation.

Comment: intra-articular trimalleolar fracture with posterolateral displacement of the distal fibula, lateral displacement of the medial malleolus, posterior displacement of the posterior malleolus and posterolateral subluxation of the talus.

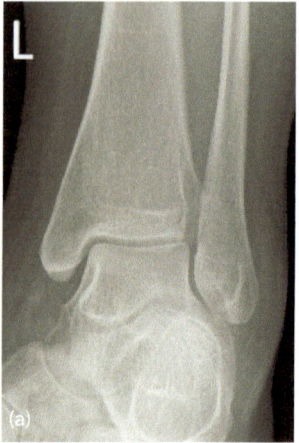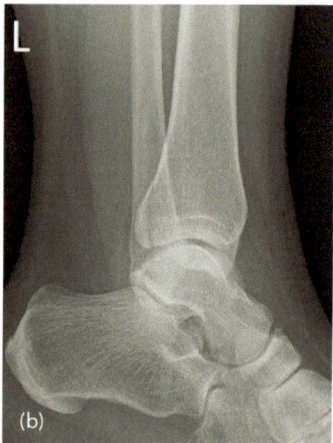

Figure 8.7 (a) AP and (b) lateral ankle images demonstrating an isolated posterior malleolus fracture.

> **Comment: isolated posterior malleolus fracture; normal mortise alignment.**

- Although calcaneal images are generally requested when an injury to the calcaneum is suspected, it is wise to assess its integrity on lateral ankle images. Calcaneal fractures may be difficult to see and there are two angles that can be measured to help determine calcaneal integrity, as demonstrated in Figure 8.1b. **Gissane's angle** is the angle created by the superior articular surface of the calcaneum and should measure between 120° and 140°. Greater than 140° indicates a fracture. **Bohler's angle** is the angle between a line from the anterior process of the calcaneum to the superior aspect of the posterior facet, and a further line from the superior aspect of the calcaneal tuberosity to the superior aspect of the posterior facet. The angle created should be between 28° and 40°. Anything less than 28° indicates a fracture. Most calcaneal fractures are intra-articular, and a computed tomography scan is often requested to fully assess the complexity of the fracture.
- Occasionally, Bohler's angle may be normal but there could still be a fracture. The trabecular pattern should be assessed, looking

for any disruption. This is commonly seen in the calcaneum as a result of a stress injury and is often associated with a sclerotic line (**Figure 8.8**).

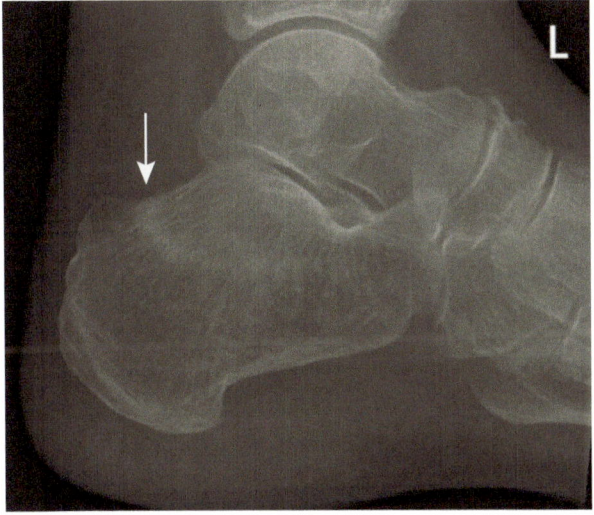

Figure 8.8 Lateral calcaneal image demonstrating a sclerotic line (vertical arrow) in keeping with a stress fracture.

- The **anterior calcaneal process** can be seen on most lateral ankle images (Figure 8.1b). This must be checked, as failure to identify a fracture in this location can lead to significant consequences and early onset of degeneration.
- An injury in the talar dome, caused by a compression mechanism or repetitive micro-trauma, is an **osteochondral fracture** (acute) or defect (chronic); both cartilage and bone are damaged, and the bone fragment may displace into the joint space. This more commonly occurs in the lateral talar dome, caused when the talus impacts with the fibula on inversion. Medial fractures are caused by impact against the medial malleolus, and the lesions tend to be deeper (**Figure 8.9**).

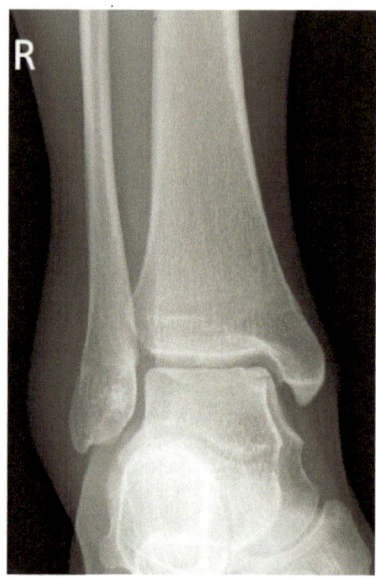

Figure 8.9 AP ankle image demonstrating irregularity in an osteochondral defect of the talar dome.

CARTILAGINOUS AREAS

- Ankle joint integrity is assessed in three ways (Figure 8.1a).

  a. The joint space around the talus should be equal medially and laterally.
  b. The talar dome and tibial plafond should be parallel.
  c. The distal tibiofibular syndesmosis should be less than 5 mm.

  If the talus has shifted, or tilted, this will cause widening within one aspect of the tibiotalar joint (**Figure 8.10a**). As the tibia and fibula complex is a ring bone equivalent, disruption of the mortise or the syndesmosis indicates a breach in the ring and a further injury should be suspected. In the absence of a visible fracture, further images are advised to exclude a fracture of the proximal fibula in an injury known as a **Maisonneuve injury** (**Figure 8.10b**).

The pain from the ankle injury can often mask the pain associated with the proximal fibula fracture. Checking alignment of the mortise will be difficult in younger children where the lateral and medial malleoli have not ossified.

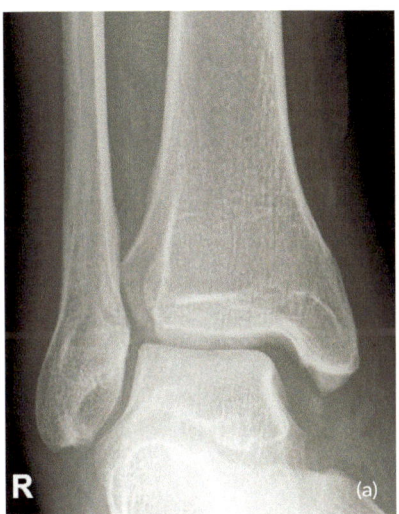 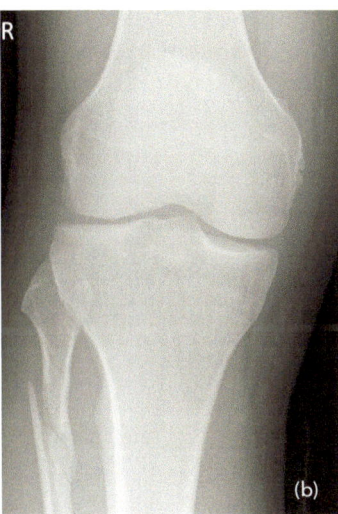

Figure 8.10 (a) AP ankle image demonstrating widening of the medial tibiotalar joint and the distal tibiofibular syndesmosis. (b) AP knee image demonstrating a fracture through the fibula neck.

- Check that the distal fibula epiphysis is normally aligned with the metaphysis on the AP ankle image of a child. Malalignment may indicate a Salter–Harris type I injury as a result of inversion. In the skeletally immature skeleton, the forces have an impact on the weaker part of the bone, which is the newly calcified bone adjacent to the metaphysis. By assessing the lateral cortex of both the metaphysis and the epiphysis, it is possible to determine if it is abnormally aligned (**Figure 8.11**). There may be soft tissue swelling and an effusion to support this diagnosis.
- As well as assessing for malalignment of the epiphysis, also check for widening of the growth plate or irregularities within the growth plate, such as fragmentation, which may indicate subtle

Salter–Harris type injuries. Look for supporting signs of injury, such as soft tissue swelling or an ankle joint effusion.

- The tarsal bones within the hindfoot and midfoot should be normally aligned. Disruption often occurs at the talonavicular and calcaneocuboid joints, causing hindfoot and midfoot separation (**Figure 8.12**) as a result of rotation on a plantar flexed foot. This joint is referred to as the Chopart joint, and injuries in this region are commonly missed.

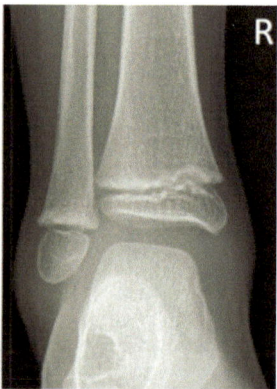

Figure 8.11 AP ankle image demonstrating displacement of the distal fibula epiphysis.

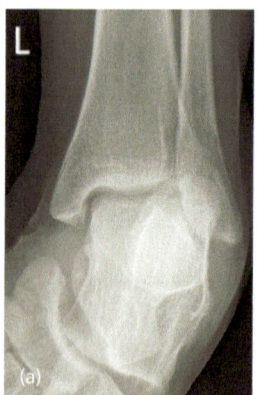 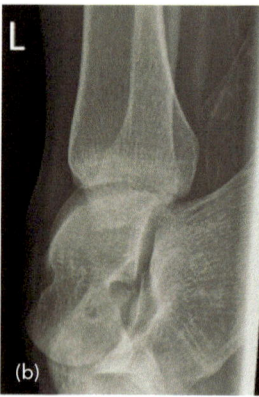

Figure 8.12 (a) AP and (b) lateral ankle images demonstrating hindfoot malalignment involving the Chopart joint.

Comment: medial subluxation at the talonavicular and calcaneocuboid joint; the mortise is normal; no fracture.

SOFT TISSUES

- Soft tissue swelling in the absence of fracture may suggest significant ligamentous injury, and this may be supported by other appearances, such as displacement of the talus within the ankle mortise.
- **Kager's fat pad** sits within Kager's triangle and indicates integrity of the Achilles tendon. This is seen as a lucent triangle posterior to the distal tibia on the lateral image (**Figure 8.13a**). The triangle will appear collapsed if the tendon is ruptured (**Figure 8.13b**).
- Look for an ankle effusion that may support a diagnosis of a Salter–Harris injury. An ankle **effusion** may be seen on the lateral image, indicated by displacement of the fat plane and increased density within the soft tissues anterior to the tibiotalar joint (**Figure 8.14**).

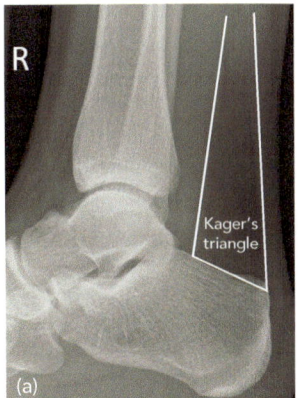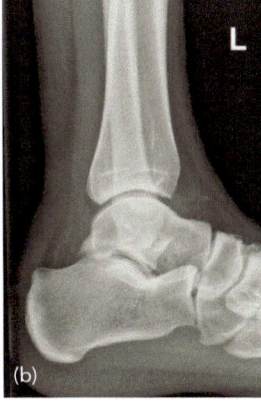

Figure 8.13 Lateral ankle images demonstrating (a) a normal Kager's triangle and (b) the collapse of the posterior border indicating rupture of the Achilles tendon.

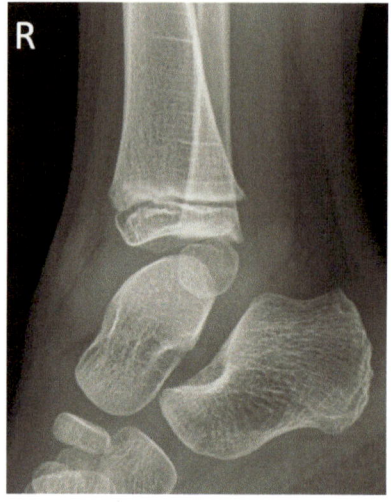

Figure 8.14 Lateral ankle image demonstrating an ankle effusion.

- There are many **accessory ossicles** visible within the soft tissues around the ankle (**Figure 8.15**), which can be mistaken for fractures. These lie in typical positions within the soft tissues and are rounded and corticated, so they should not be mistaken for a fracture fragment.

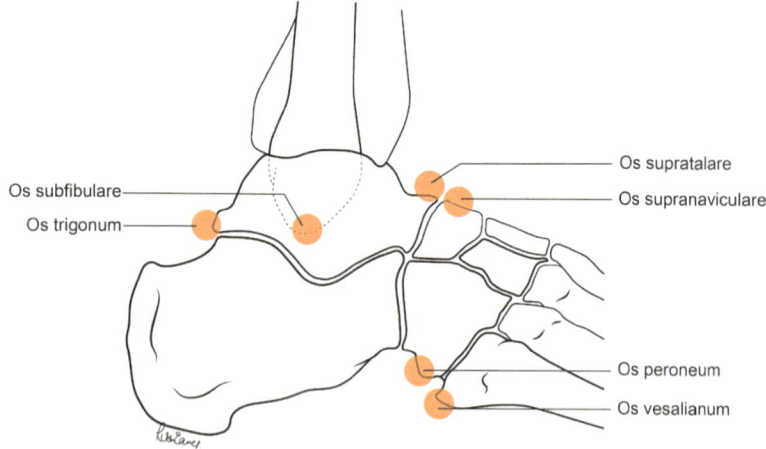

Os subfibulare

Os trigonum

Os supratalare

Os supranaviculare

Os peroneum

Os vesalianum

Figure 8.15 Locations of some of the accessory ossicles around the ankle joint.

CHAPTER SUMMARY

- Ankle integrity is assessed by checking that the tibial plafond and talus are parallel on the AP image and that the syndesmosis is not greater than 5 mm.
- Gissane's and Bohler's angles can be assessed to determine calcaneal integrity. Gissane's angle should be 120–140°. Anything greater than 140° may indicate a fracture. Bohler's angle should be 28–40°. Anything less than 28° may indicate a fracture.

REFERENCE

1. Han, S.M., Wu, T.H., Wen, J.X., Wang, Y., Cao, L., Wu, W.J. et al. Radiographic analysis of adult ankle fractures using combined Danis-Weber and Lauge-Hansen classification systems. *Scientific Reports* 2020;**10**:7655.

9. KNEE AND DISTAL FEMUR

This chapter will focus on evaluation of the knee, as femoral fractures are often easy to identify due to the displacement caused by the pull of strong muscles. The knee is the largest joint in the body, and it is supported by strong ligaments, so tibiofemoral dislocations are rare. Patella dislocations, however, do occur, more commonly in adolescents, and can be either traumatic or because of a developmental anomaly. Bony injury around the knee tends to involve the tibial plateau and fractures can be subtle. Soft tissues should be assessed for **effusion** or **lipohaemarthrosis**, with the latter always being associated with a fracture. Abnormalities associated with common mechanisms of injury are found in **Table 9.1**.

The knee is often one of the first joints to develop degenerative disease and to require replacement surgery. Abnormalities associated with a prosthesis, such as periprosthetic fracture, loosening or infection, should always be considered.

There are few normal variants around the knee, but an important one is the child's tibial tuberosity, which can develop from multiple centres, mimicking Osgood–Schlatter's disease – apophysitis of the

Table 9.1 Common mechanisms of injury and associated abnormalities in the knee and femur.

Mechanism	Typical abnormality
Twisting injury	Avulsion of the tibial spine
	Patella dislocation
	Femoral fracture
	Segond fracture from the proximal tibia
Direct impact	Patella or femoral fracture
	Salter–Harris type II distal femur fracture
Valgus (lateral) or varus (medial) strain	Tibial plateau fracture
	Patella dislocation
Hyperextension	Tibial tuberosity avulsion

tibial tubercle. Without point tenderness, this appearance is a normal variant.

Building on the ABCs method of evaluation, as introduced in Chapter 1, and assuming that adequacy has been checked, **Table 9.2** includes the more specific checks related to evaluation of the knee, such as evaluation of soft tissues. **Figure 9.1** demonstrates normal anteroposterior (AP) and lateral knee images, summarising these additional checks for knee images, which will be discussed in more detail in this chapter.

Table 9.2 Summary of the systematic checks to be made when evaluating the knee.

Focus	Points to consider
Bones	Pay particular attention to the tibial spines and tibial plateau, as fractures here can be subtle.
	Identification of the medial and lateral femoral condyles on the lateral image can be difficult; however, there are two distinct anatomical structures that can help. The adductor tubercle is on the medial condyle and the femoral notch is on the lateral condyle.
Cartilaginous areas	The articular surfaces at the tibiofemoral joint should be congruent with no more than a 5 mm difference between the outer margins of the distal femur and the proximal tibia on a reasonably positioned AP image.
	The patella should be centrally located on the AP image. When it subluxes or dislocates, it generally shifts laterally, as the lateral condyle is shallower than the medial condyle.
	Loose bodies may be present within the joint spaces, and these can cause locking of the knee joint.
	Calcification within the meniscus may be present. This is a precursor to degenerative disease or other pathology.
Soft tissues	On the lateral image, the suprapatellar region is important, as this is the site for an effusion that is caused when there is a build-up of excessive synovial fluid within the suprapatellar bursa. Effusions are assessed by measuring the distance between the pre-femoral fat pad and the quadriceps tendon, which should be no greater than 10 mm.
	A lipohaemarthrosis, comprising blood and fat from within the marrow, may also be present within the bursa. This indicates that a fracture is present.
	Bulging of the medial and lateral soft tissues may indicate injury to the collateral ligaments.

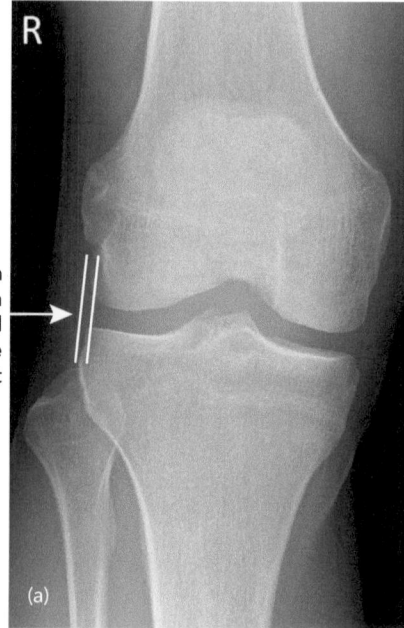

<5 mm difference in tibiofemoral outer condyle alignment

Figure 9.1 (a) AP and (b) lateral knee images demonstrating the checks that are unique to this area.

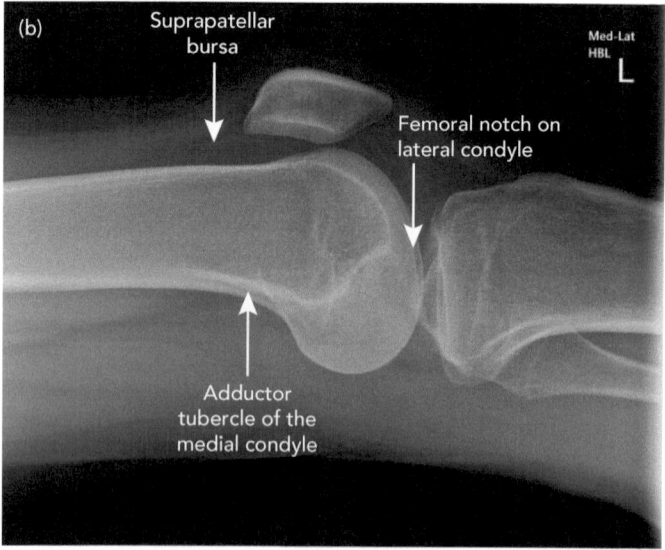

(b) Suprapatellar bursa

Femoral notch on lateral condyle

Med-Lat HBL
L

Adductor tubercle of the medial condyle

BONES

- Femoral shaft fractures are typically easy to see, but if a femoral shaft fracture is identified in a very young child, then the mechanism of injury needs to be checked to exclude an injury caused by **physical abuse** (see Chapter 13).
- The most fractured bone around the knee joint is the patella, and this can be a simple transverse fracture or a comminuted fracture. The mechanism of injury is direct impact and/or indirect forces causing knee flexion with the quadriceps muscle contracted. The fracture can have significant distraction due to the pull of the strong thigh muscles (**Figure 9.2**). Differentiation is needed between a fractured patella and a **bipartite patella** in which the patella ossifies from two centres that do not fuse. If there are more than two parts, this is a multipartite patella. The additional ossification centres are normally visible in the upper outer quadrant of the patella, are well corticated and do not recreate the normal shape when closely aligned with the patella (**Figure 9.3**).

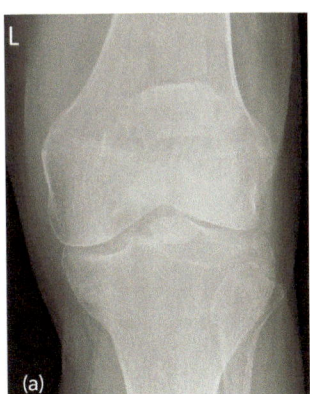

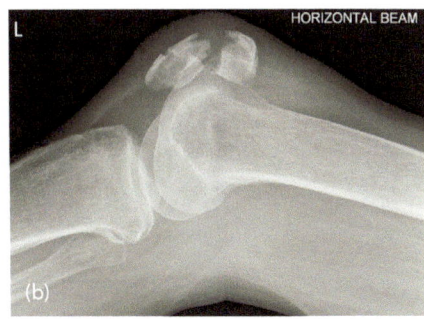

Figure 9.2 (a) AP and (b) lateral knee images demonstrating a comminuted fracture of the patella.

Comment: **there is a distracted comminuted fracture of the patella.**

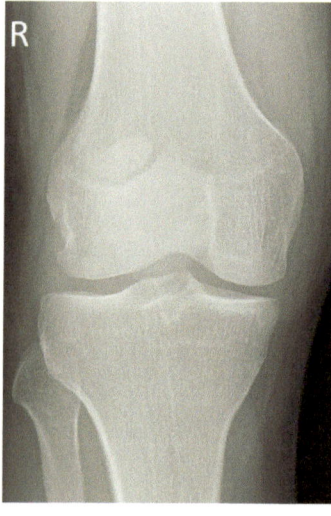

Figure 9.3 AP knee image demonstrating a bipartite patella.

- **Tibial plateau fractures** can be extremely comminuted or subtle. A sclerotic line below the tibial plateau on the AP or lateral image may indicate a fracture (**Figure 9.4**). The mechanism of injury is a varus or valgus force while weight bearing.

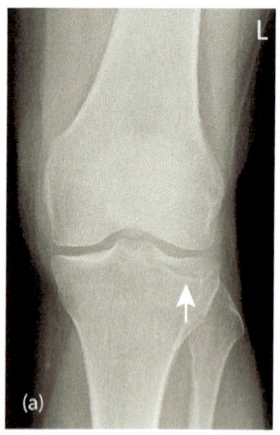

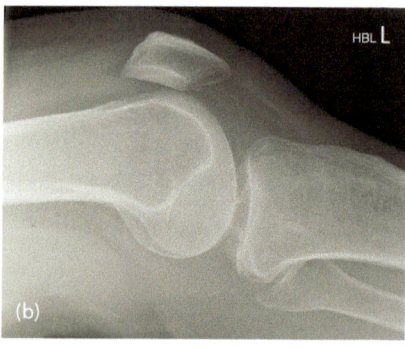

Figure 9.4 (a) AP and (b) lateral knee images demonstrating subtle subarticular sclerosis in keeping with a tibial plateau fracture.

Comment: fracture of the lateral tibial plateau.

- Irregularity in the femoral cortex may represent an **osteochondral lesion** in which the articular cartilage and underlying bone are damaged. More commonly, this is seen in the lateral aspect of the medial femoral condyle (**Figure 9.5**), but occasionally it occurs in the lateral condyle. In an acute osteochondral fracture, there will be a history of trauma, usually a twisting mechanism while weight bearing, and the lesion can occur in either condyle. It is most common in adolescents who take part in sporting activities such as football, and there is an association with patella dislocation and anterior cruciate ligament rupture.[1] A chronic condition, **osteochondritis dissecans**, has similar appearances and is caused by repetitive micro-trauma with the blood supply being disrupted to a small piece of bone. In both acute and chronic injuries, the bony fragment and adjacent cartilage may become loose and lodge within the joint space, causing locking of the knee or the knee giving way.

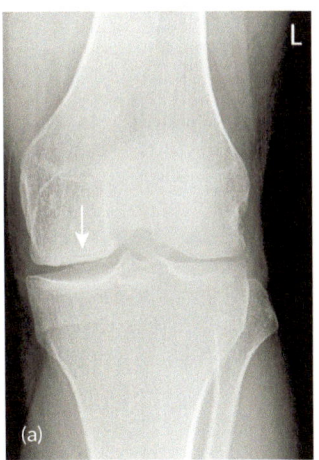
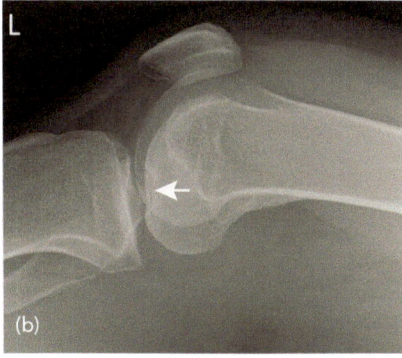

Figure 9.5 (a) AP and (b) lateral knee images demonstrating an osteochondral lesion in the medial femoral condyle.

Comment: **osteochondral lesion in the medial femoral condyle with an effusion.**

■ Older patients may have a **joint replacement** *in situ*, and it is
important to look for problems associated with it. A **periprosthetic
fracture** can occur from relatively minor trauma, as the prosthesis
acts as a pivot, with the fracture occurring at the most proximal or
distal aspect (**Figure 9.6a**). The prosthesis may start to loosen, and
close attention should be paid to the junction of the bone and the
implant. There should be close contact without any lucency around
the prosthesis. A lucency of greater than 2 mm is suspicious for
loosening (Figure 9.6b), but it is important to look at images taken
immediately after surgery to differentiate between loosening and
a non-pathological cause of lucency associated with surgery. In the
latter, a fibrous layer may develop between the prosthesis and the
bone, but this will have a subtle sclerotic margin and be less than
2 mm.

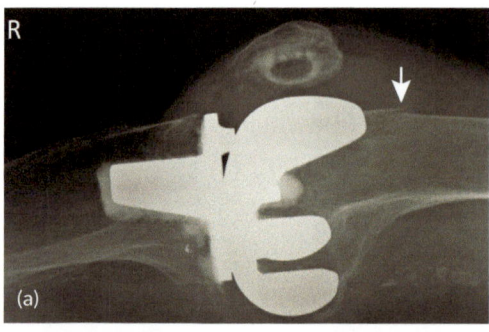

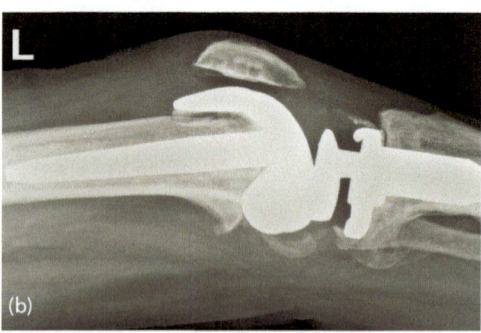

Figure 9.6 Lateral knee images demonstrating (a) a distal femoral periprosthetic
fracture and (b) loosening of the femoral component.

CARTILAGINOUS AREAS

- The knee joint is one of the body's largest weight-bearing joints; it suffers from the stresses applied and commonly degenerates in later life. This manifests as a reduction in the tibiofemoral joint, with other associated signs of degeneration (see Chapter 15).
- Alignment at the tibiofemoral joint is checked by assessing alignment at the articular margins of the condyles (Figure 9.1a). Occasionally, the tibial plateau may extend beyond the articular surface of the femoral condyle. Providing that it is within 5 mm, this is acceptable. Greater than 5 mm indicates an abnormality, and the most common cause of this is a tibial plateau fracture or degenerative malalignment.
- While the tibiofemoral joint does occasionally dislocate, more common dislocations involve the patellofemoral joint. The mechanism of injury is **valgus** (lateral) stress put on a flexed knee causing it to twist or a direct blow to the medial aspect of the patella. Due to the shallow lateral femoral condyle and the pull of the quadriceps muscle, the patella dislocates laterally (**Figure 9.7**) and is the most common injury in a child's knee.[2]

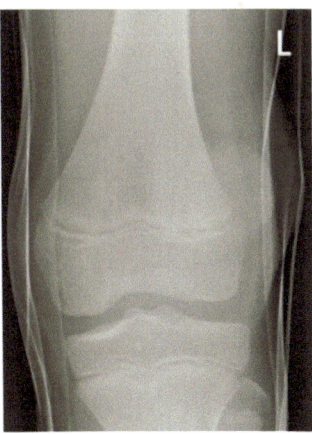

Figure 9.7 AP knee image demonstrating lateral displacement of the patella indicating a patella dislocation.

SOFT TISSUES

- The meniscal cartilages and the ligaments that stabilise the knee are often injured, but these cannot be seen on an X-ray image and require a magnetic resonance imaging scan to enable a diagnosis.
- Soft tissue signs around the knee joint are extremely important. Patients may have an **effusion**. This is an increase in the fluid within the joint and is seen within the suprapatellar bursa on a lateral image (**Figure 9.8a**). It is assessed by measuring the distance between the pre-femoral fat pad and the quadriceps tendon, which should be no greater than 10 mm (**Figure 9.8b**). An effusion can occur without a fracture being present.

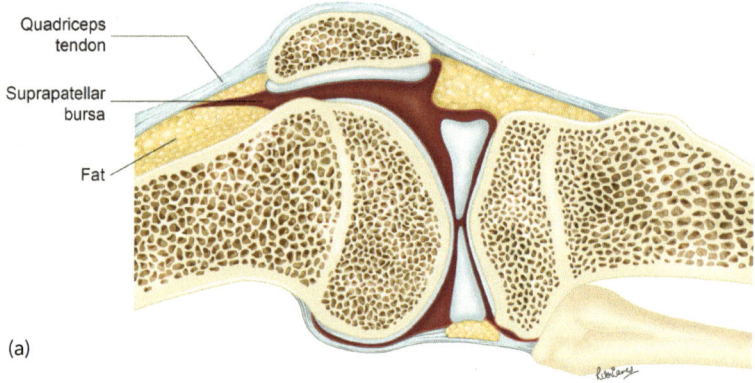

Quadriceps tendon

Suprapatellar bursa

Fat

(a)

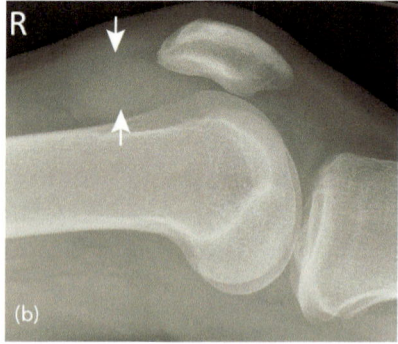

(b)

Figure 9.8 (a) Knee anatomy demonstrating the location of the suprapatellar bursa. (b) Horizontal beam lateral knee image demonstrating an effusion.

- A **lipohaemarthrosis** is a type of effusion and is highly likely to be associated with fracture. This is seen when the bone marrow escapes through an intra-articular fracture into the joint. The fatty marrow separates from the watery blood and appears as a clear line of separation within the joint capsule on a horizontal beam lateral knee image (**Figure 9.9**). More than half of tibial plateau fractures will not have a lipohaemarthrosis but will have the appearance of an effusion or haemarthrosis instead. In addition, a lipohaemarthrosis may not be apparent in a patient who has not been supine with their leg extended prior to imaging.
- Around 40% of patients will have a small, rounded accessory ossicle behind the knee called a **fabella**. This is a normal variant, identified by its location and classical accessory ossicle features. However, if a fragment of bone is seen elsewhere within the soft tissues, a fracture should be considered.

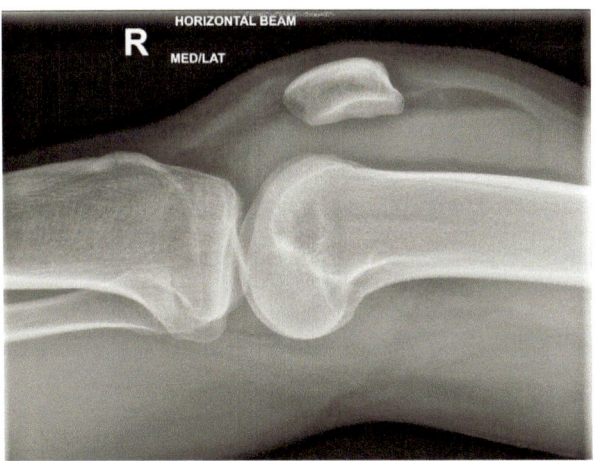

Figure 9.9 Lateral knee image demonstrating a lipohaemarthrosis.

- A **Segond fracture** presents as a small fragment of bone adjacent to the lateral tibial condyle and it may be missed if there is slight rotation on the AP image (**Figure 9.10a**). The mechanism of injury is medial stress with internal rotation and is usually a result of a sporting injury. There is a high association with meniscal injury and a very high association with anterior cruciate ligament rupture.[3] The fracture is extracapsular, so may not be associated with an effusion or lipohaemarthrosis (**Figure 9.10b**), although there will likely be extensive soft tissue swelling. Rarely, an avulsion fracture will occur from the medial condyle with rupture of the posterior cruciate ligament, and this is a reverse Segond fracture.

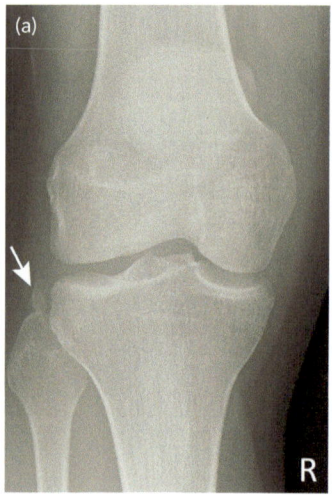
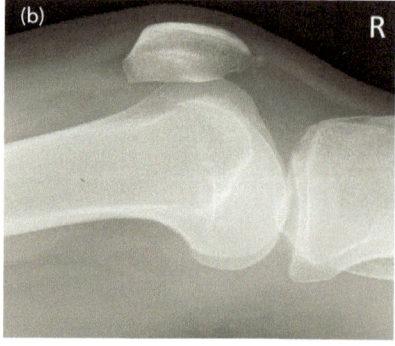

Figure 9.10 (a) AP knee image demonstrating an avulsion fracture from the lateral tibial plateau in keeping with a Segond fracture. (b) Lateral knee image with no associated significant effusion or lipohaemarthrosis; note the small accessory ossicle inferior to the patella with classical accessory ossicle features.

Comment: there is an avulsion fracture from the lateral tibial condyle.

CHAPTER SUMMARY

- There can be subtle fractures around the knee joint, and good technique and careful evaluation are key in identifying these.
- The articular surfaces at the tibiofemoral joint should be no more than a 5 mm difference between the outer margins.
- The patella should be centrally located on the AP image.
- Patella dislocation is generally laterally.
- Effusions and lipohaemarthrosis can be found in the suprapatellar region.

REFERENCES

1. Kuhle, J., Angele, P., Balcarek, P., Eichinger, M., Feucht, M., Haasper, C. et al. Treatment of osteochondral fractures of the knee: a meta-analysis of available scientific evidence. *International Orthopaedics* 2013;**37**(12):2385–2394.
2. Jaquith, B.P. and Parikh, S.N. Predictors of recurrent patellar instability in children and adolescents after first-time dislocation. *Journal of Pediatric Orthopaedics* 2017;**37**(7):484–490.
3. Arneja, S.S., Furey, M.J., Alvarez, C.M. and Reilly, C.W. Segond fractures. *Sports Health* 2010;**2**(5):437–439.

10. PELVIS AND HIP

The pelvis and hips are inextricably linked, and whether pelvis imaging is obtained for femoral neck fractures or pelvic injuries, it is essential that the whole image is assessed. The most common traumatic finding on a pelvis image is a femoral neck fracture, with many occurring in older people because of osteoporosis. Injuries to the femoral neck in children involve the proximal femoral epiphysis, as the forces from the injury have an impact on the weakest part of the bone. Additionally, children may present to the Emergency Department with an atraumatic limp or hip pain, and knowing the radiological appearances of the more common pathologies will assist in providing a comment.

The pelvis is a ring bone, having the main pelvic ring and two obturator rings. An abnormality in one part may lead to a further abnormality within the ring, which could be another fracture or widening of the symphysis pubis or sacroiliac joints. It is important to recognise every component of the injury, so that the classification, as either **stable** or **unstable**, can be made by the referring clinician.

In addition to the normal process of evaluation, the pelvic lines need to be checked, as they are useful in assessing for fractures of the acetabulum, for example. Abnormalities associated with common mechanisms of injury are found in **Table 10.1**, and common paediatric hip pathologies presenting with atraumatic hip pain are listed in **Table 10.2**.

Table 10.1 Common mechanisms of injury and associated abnormalities in the pelvis and hip.

Mechanism	Typical abnormality
Anteroposterior compression force	Sacroiliac/symphysis pubis diastasis Fracture involving the pelvic bones
Lateral compression force	Pubic ramus fracture Sacral fracture Fracture involving the iliac wings
Muscle contraction	Apophysis avulsion
Vertical shearing	Pubic ramus fracture Sacroiliac diastasis Fracture of the iliac wing
Fall	Fracture to the neck of the femur
Fall onto the lateral aspect of the hip	Greater trochanter fracture
Road traffic collision: driver/ passenger	Hip dislocation

Table 10.2 Differential diagnoses for atraumatic hip pain in children.

Age	Differential diagnosis
0–3 years	Congenital or developmental dysplasia of the hip
4–9 years	Legg–Calve–Perthes disease
10 years – fusion	Slipped upper femoral epiphysis (SUFE)
Any age	Fracture Infection Physical abuse

Building on the ABCs method of evaluation (see Chapter 1), and assuming that adequacy has been checked, **Table 10.3** includes the more specific checks related to evaluation of the pelvis and hip, such as lines of Judet. **Figure 10.1** demonstrates a normal anteroposterior (AP) pelvis and a lateral hip image, summarising these additional checks for pelvis and hip images, which will be discussed in more detail in this chapter.

Table 10.3 Summary of systematic checks to be made when evaluating the pelvis and hip.

Focus	Points to consider
Bones	Trabecula lines are distinctive due to the lines of stress, and disruption must raise concerns for a fracture (see Figure 10.2).
	Shenton's line helps in identifying a fracture of the femoral neck.
	A subchondral lucency, associated with osteonecrosis, may be seen in the femoral head.
	Six lines of Judet help to identify acetabular injuries (see Figure 10.8).
	Sacral arcuate lines should be intact (see Figure 10.10).
	The coccyx should be assessed if it is visible.
	The lumbar spine should be checked.
	Any prosthesis should be checked for adverse features.
Cartilaginous areas	The acetabular articular surface should be congruous with the femoral head indicating normal articulation.
	Klein's line allows alignment of the proximal femoral epiphysis with the femoral neck to be checked (see Figure 10.15).
	The sacroiliac joints and symphysis pubis should not be widened.
Soft tissues	Apophyseal avulsions may result in a bone fragment being seen within the soft tissues (see Figure 10.12).
	The gluteal fat stripe should be checked in children, as this may indicate an effusion due to irritable hip (see Figure 10.17).

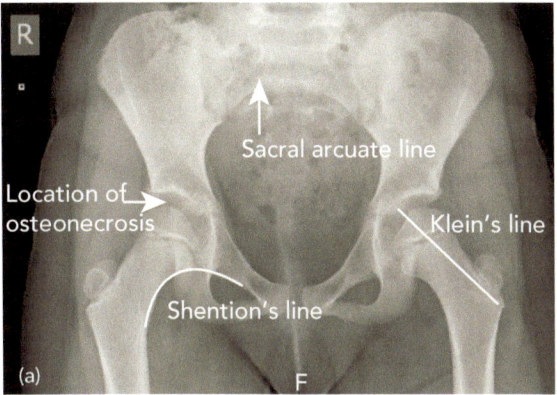

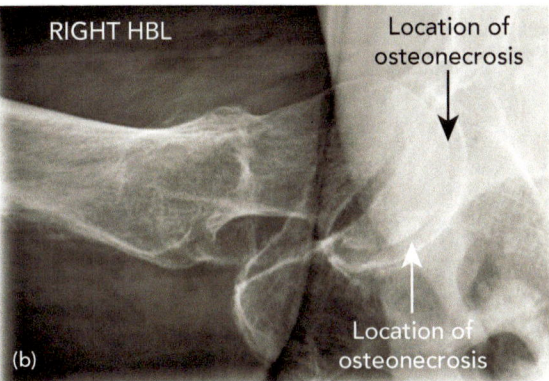

Figure 10.1 (a) AP paediatric pelvis and (b) horizontal beam lateral adult hip images demonstrating the checks that are unique to this area.

BONES

■ Mechanical forces on the proximal femora result in a distinctive trabecular pattern (**Figure 10.2**), which can be disrupted in subtle fractures. The pattern of trabecula lines leaves a weak area (Ward's triangle) with stress fractures occurring here.

- Femoral neck fractures are classified as intracapsular and extracapsular.
- **Intracapsular fractures** involve the proximal aspect of the femoral neck and the femoral head and may be treated with a **dynamic hip screw** (DHS) in younger patients or with a **hemi-arthroplasty** in older patients. There is a high incidence of **osteonecrosis** due to interruption of the blood supplying the femoral head. The categories of intracapsular fractures are as follows.
  - **Subcapital** fractures are often subtle and seen as a cortical breach at the junction of the femoral head and neck (**Figure 10.3a**). **Shenton's line**, drawn along the inferior femoral neck and the inferior border of the superior pubic ramus, should be seen with a small part of the femoral head extending below this (Figure 10.1a). If the femoral head does not extend below, then this is a marker for a subcapital fracture in an adult or a slipped upper femoral epiphysis in a child.
  - **Transcervical** fractures occur across the middle of the femoral neck (**Figure 10.3b**).
  - **Basicervical** fractures occur through the base of the femoral neck and may be intracapsular or extracapsular (**Figure 10.3c**).

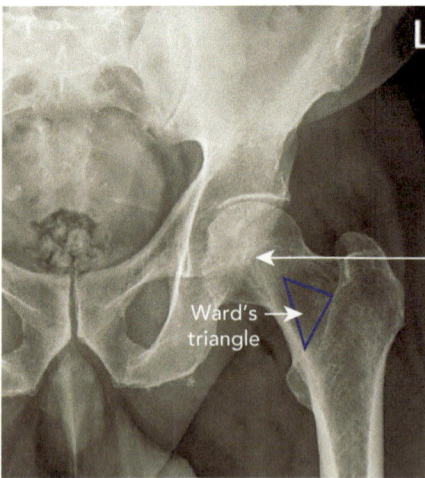

Lines of mechanical stress

Ward's triangle

Figure 10.2 AP hip image demonstrating lines of mechanical stress and Ward's triangle.

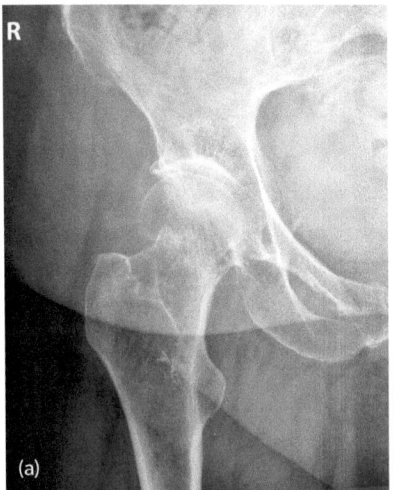
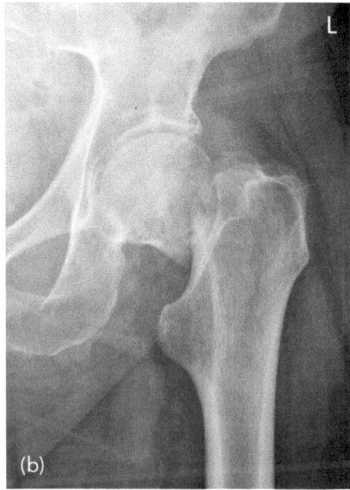
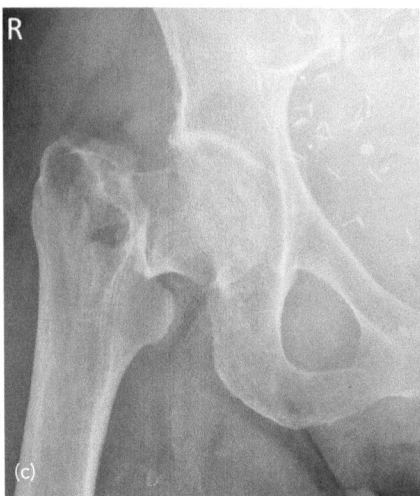

Figure 10.3 AP hip images demonstrating (a) a subcapital fracture, (b) a transcervical fracture and (c) a basicervical fracture; note also the metallic artefacts from previous abdominal surgery.

- **Extracapsular fractures** are in the region of the trochanters, with fractures extending from greater to lesser trochanters. The categories of extracapsular fractures are as follows.

    - **Intertrochanteric** fractures extend from lesser to greater trochanters (**Figure 10.4a**).
    - **Pertrochanteric** fractures are similar to intertrochanteric fractures, but the fracture is comminuted with avulsion of the lesser trochanter (**Figure 10.4b**).

    Extracapsular fractures are treated with a DHS or a proximal femoral nailing anti-rotation device.

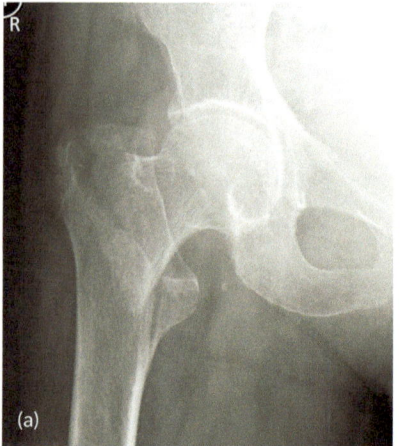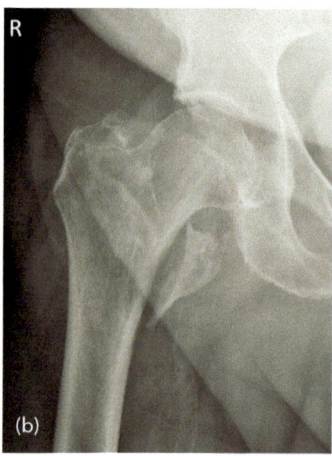

Figure 10.4 AP hip images demonstrating (a) an intertrochanteric fracture and (b) a pertrochanteric fracture.

- Fractures distal to the trochanters, **subtrochanteric fractures**, tend to be pathological, and it may be beneficial to obtain full femoral images to look for pathological lesions.
- If there is surgical metalwork on an image, it is important to look for signs of **loosening**, which appear as a lucency around the metalwork (see Figure 9.6b) or a **periprosthetic fracture** (**Figure 10.5**). In addition, there may be a hemi-arthroplasty dislocation (discussed later in this chapter) or infection (discussed in Chapter 16).

- Close evaluation of the femoral head may reveal a subchondral lucency, often referred to as a crescent sign. This is the early sign of **osteonecrosis** and is caused by disruption to the blood supply in this area. It generally occurs following injury, but it can also be atraumatic. As it progresses, it leads to increased sclerosis and deformity within the bony contour of the femoral head (**Figure 10.6**).

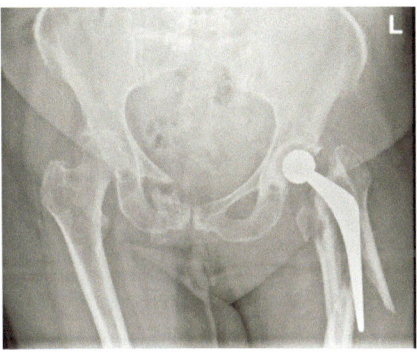

Figure 10.5 AP pelvis image demonstrating a left periprosthetic fracture and non-union of right pubic rami fractures.

Comment: comminuted periprosthetic fracture of the left femur; old right pubic rami fractures.

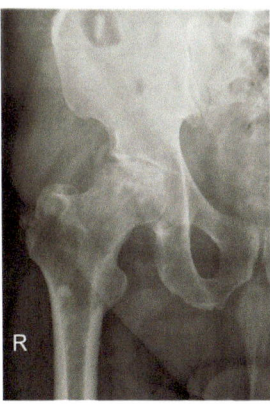

Figure 10.6 AP hip image demonstrating osteonecrosis of the right femoral head.

Comment: osteonecrosis of the right femoral head.

- Osteonecrosis in a child is usually associated with **Legg–Calve– Perthes disease** (commonly shortened to Perthes disease). The child, usually between the ages of 4 and 9 years, will present with limping and pain in the affected hip. The subchondral lucency is initially seen on the turned lateral hip image (**Figure 10.7a**) and may not be seen on an AP pelvis image at the initial presentation. If the limp persists, repeat imaging will show the lucency on the AP image (**Figure 10.7b**). Over time, flattening of the femoral head will occur.

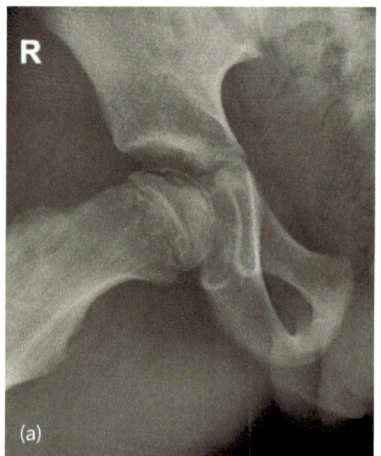 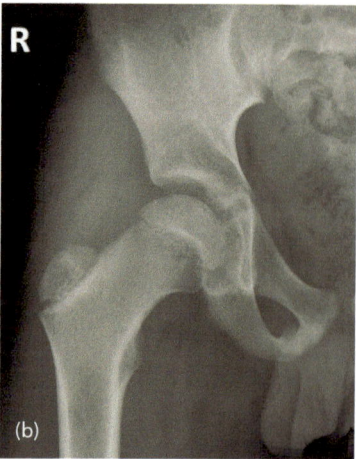

Figure 10.7 Subchondral lucency seen on (a) a turned lateral hip image and (b) an AP hip image demonstrating Perthes disease.

> **Comment: irregularity in the right femoral head.**

- Acetabular fractures are identified by assessing the **six lines of Judet (Figure 10.8)**. These are the:

1. acetabular roof indicating the superior acetabulum;
2. anterior acetabular rim indicating the anterior acetabulum;
3. posterior acetabular rim indicating the posterior acetabulum;
4. teardrop sign indicating the medial acetabular wall;

5. iliopectineal line indicating the anterior column;
6. ilioischial line indicating the posterior column.

If there is a breach in any of these lines, then an acetabular fracture is indicated (**Figure 10.9**).

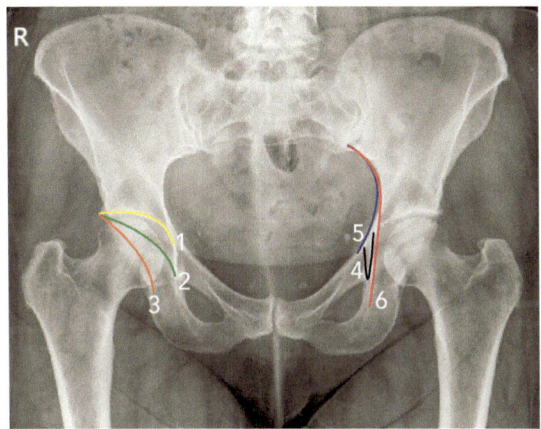

Figure 10.8 AP pelvis image demonstrating Judet lines.

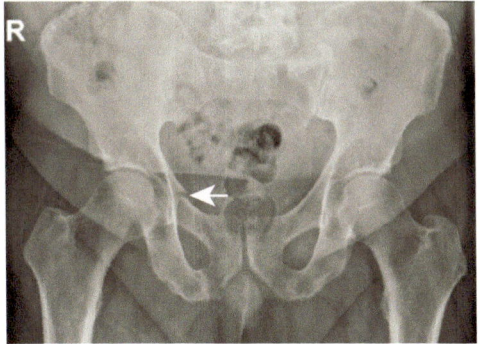

Figure 10.9 AP pelvis image demonstrating a breach in the iliopectineal line.

Comment: fracture of the right superior pubic ramus (anterior acetabular column).

- Checking the **sacral arcuate lines** will help to identify sacral fractures (**Figure 10.10**), but they may be obscured by overlying bowel contents. There should be no breaches of these lines, and they should be bilaterally equal.

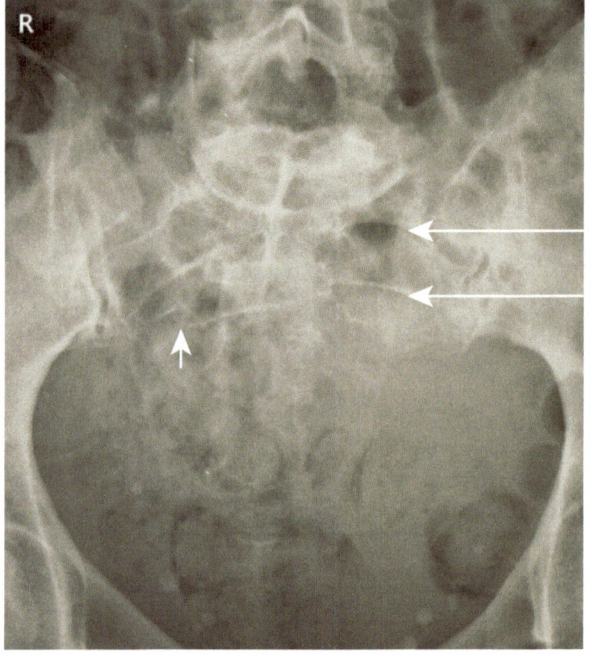

Normal sacral arcuate lines

Figure 10.10 AP sacrum image demonstrating irregularity in the right sacral arcuate lines indicating a fracture of the right sacral ala.

Comment: fracture of the right sacral ala.

- The iliac wing can fracture in a simple fall in older people (**Figure 10.11**). Remember that the pelvis is a ring bone, so look for the second abnormality, which may be a further fracture or disruption of the symphysis pubis or sacroiliac joints. An isolated iliac wing fracture does not involve the pelvic ring if it does not extend to the iliopectineal line.
- The visualised lumbar spine should be checked. A fracture of the transverse process of L5 may be a sign that there is a sacral fracture or diastasis/dislocation of the sacroiliac joint.
- There are several **apophyses** in the immature skeleton that can be avulsed (**Figure 10.12**), generally during a sporting activity, which can lead to forceful muscle contractions. The following are some of the more common avulsion sites.

  - The greater trochanter appears around 3 years of age.
  - The lesser trochanter appears around 12 years of age.
  - The iliac crest, anterior superior iliac spine (ASIS) and anterior inferior iliac spine (AIIS) appear around 14 years of age.
  - The ischial tuberosity appears around 16 years of age.

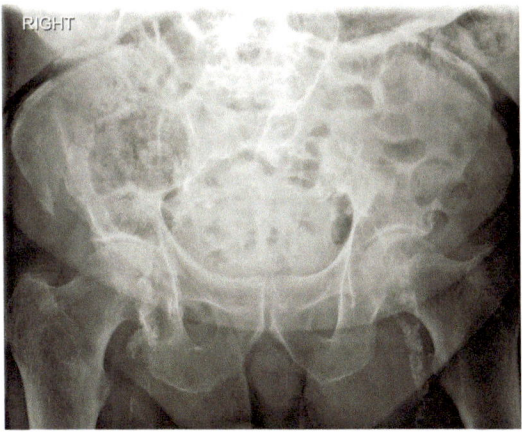

Figure 10.11 AP pelvis image demonstrating a fracture of the right iliac wing.

Comment: **isolated right iliac wing fracture.**

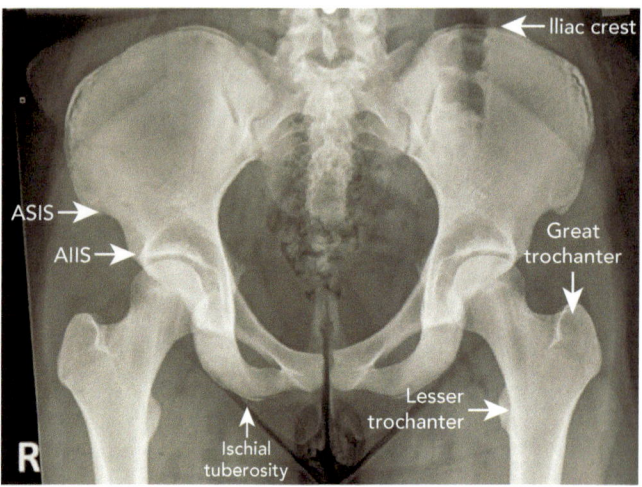

Figure 10.12 AP pelvis image demonstrating avulsion sites in a paediatric pelvis.

CARTILAGINOUS AREAS

- The articular surface of the acetabulum should be congruous with the femoral head indicating normal hip articulation. Hip dislocations, with or without a prosthesis, are generally obvious to see on an AP pelvis image. As well as occurring following trauma, a **dislocated prosthesis (Figure 10.13)** may occur without trauma in the early post-operative period before the hip capsule and supporting muscles have had time to repair fully.

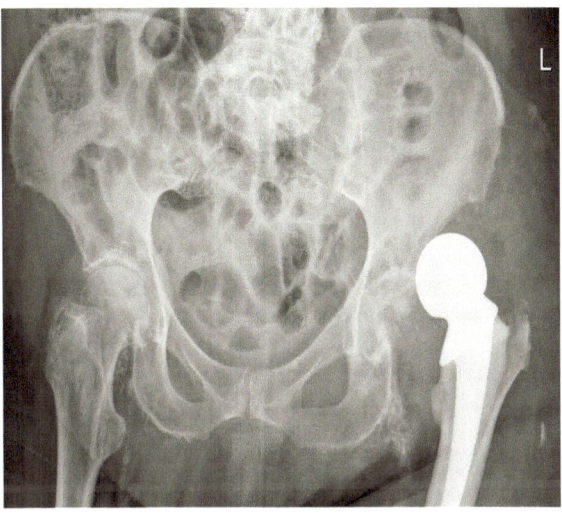

Figure 10.13 AP pelvis image demonstrating superior dislocation of the left prosthesis.

> **Comment: superior dislocation of left hip prosthesis.**

- Dislocations occur in children but are usually limited to younger children with **developmental dysplasia of the hip** (DDH) or **congenital dislocation of the hip** (CDH). Post-natal screening tests usually identify this condition; however, a child may present with a limp or delayed walking. The femoral head and/or acetabulum fail to develop normally, and the femoral head migrates superolaterally (**Figure 10.14**). Early diagnosis is key to effective treatment, as the dysplasia causes inadequate articulation leading to a dysfunctional joint, which undergoes changes to compensate for the abnormality. This will lead to disability and early degenerative disease.

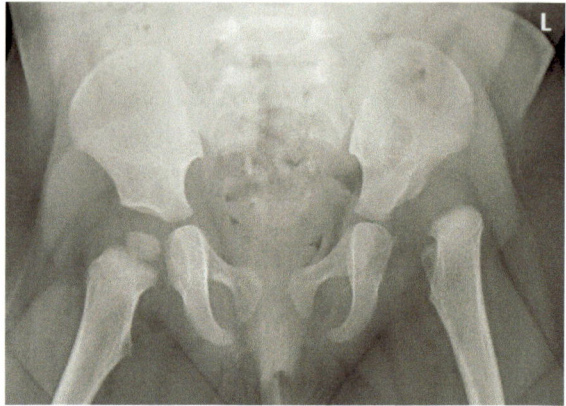

Figure 10.14 AP pelvis image demonstrating abnormal development of the left acetabulum and femoral head leading to dislocation.

Comment: superolateral dislocation of the left femur.

- The most important cartilaginous area in the hip of a child over the age of 10 years is the proximal femoral epiphysis. A **slipped proximal (or upper) femoral epiphysis (SUFE)** can be acute, due to excessive force applied to the hip joint, or chronic, generally in obese children who may present with no history of injury. The femoral heads should be the same height, and Klein's line should pass through the epiphysis (**Figure 10.15**). However, as the epiphysis slips, it moves backwards and medially so it appears shorter on the AP image, and Klein's line will not pass through a part of the epiphysis (**Figure 10.16a**). A lateral projection will show a SUFE in the early stages due to the posterior movement of the femoral epiphysis (**Figure 10.16b**).

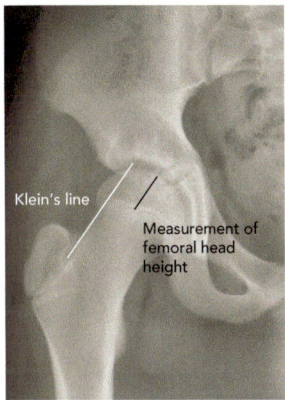

Figure 10.15 AP pelvis image demonstrating Klein's line and measurement of the height of the femoral head.

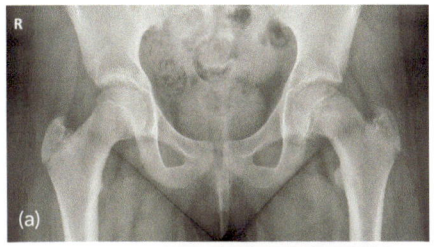

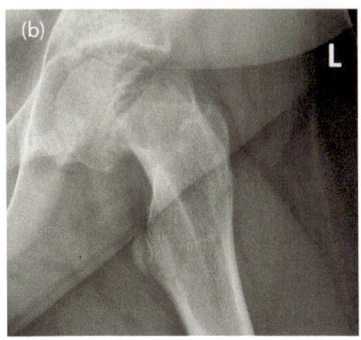

Figure 10.16 (a) AP pelvis and (b) lateral hip images demonstrating a left SUFE.

Comment: **left SUFE.**

SOFT TISSUES

- An acute atraumatic limp between the ages of 3 and 6 years may be caused by **irritable hip** or by transient synovitis in a child who has recently had a viral infection. Ultrasound is the modality of choice for this diagnosis, but, if imaging is performed, the **gluteal fat stripe (Figure 10.17a)** may be bulging and there may be widening of the medial joint space caused by an effusion. However, imaging is not as reliable as ultrasound, which will show increased fluid within the joint (**Figure 10.17b**). This is a self-limiting condition and will resolve in most cases. Failure to resolve may indicate Perthes disease or other bony pathology.
- Various soft tissue calcifications may be visible.

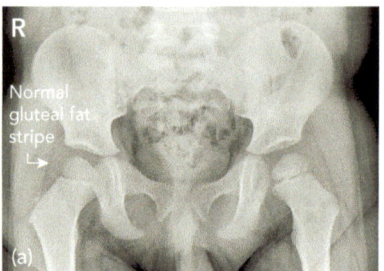 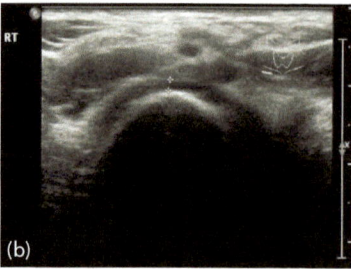

Figure 10.17 (a) AP pelvis image demonstrating normal right gluteal fat stripe. (b) Ultrasound scan of the left hip demonstrating increased fluid in keeping with an effusion.

- Calcification of the arteries (**atherosclerosis**) is most often seen in the abdominal aorta and iliac arteries (**Figure 10.18**). Venous calcifications (**phleboliths**) are small, round areas of calcification in the lower pelvis (Figure 10.18). These can be mistaken for ureteric or bladder calculi. There are subtle differences but, for the purpose of commenting, unless the patient presents with symptoms of renal colic, this appearance is likely to represent phleboliths and does not warrant inclusion in a comment, unless local procedures indicate otherwise.

- **Stones** may be visible in the gallbladder. This does not necessarily require an urgent report, but inclusion in the comment may be helpful to the referring clinician.
- **Fibroids** are calcifications in or around the uterus and are irregular in appearance (**Figure 10.19**). They are benign and do not need to be included in a comment.

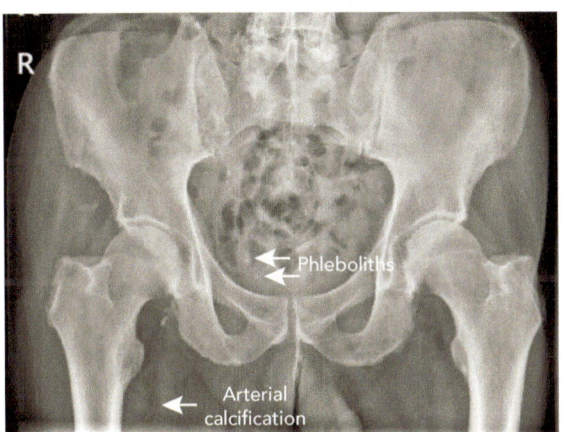

Figure 10.18 AP pelvis image demonstrating areas of calcification.

Comment: no fracture on this single image.

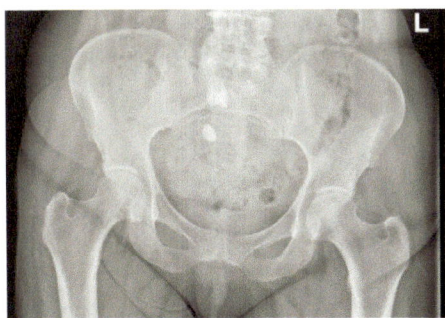

Figure 10.19 AP pelvis image demonstrating fibroids.

Comment: no fracture on this single image.

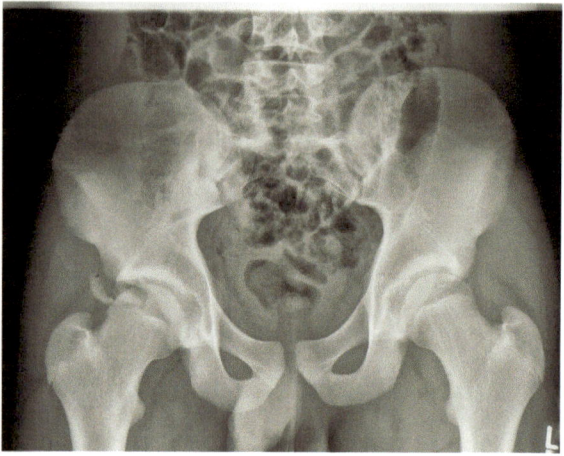

Figure 10.20 AP pelvis image demonstrating a fragment in the soft tissues adjacent to the right AIIS.

Comment: avulsion of right AIIS.

- Calcifications may be related to **avulsed apophyses** as discussed earlier and seen in **Figure 10.20**.
- As the whole image should be evaluated, it is important to look at the visualised **abdominal contents**. For commenting, it is not important to be able to interpret the appearances of pathologies, but it is important to know when these should be expedited for urgent report.

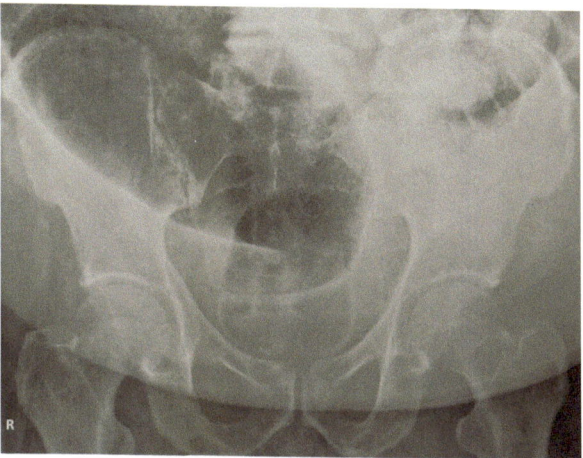

Figure 10.21 AP pelvis image demonstrating dilated bowel.

> **Comment: no fracture seen on the AP image. Dilated bowel. Image expedited for urgent report.**

- The small and large intestine will be visible through the presence of gas and faeces and, in most patients, will have normal appearances. If the bowel appears dilated (**Figure 10.21**) and prior imaging has not identified an abnormality, the image must be expedited for urgent report. See Chapter 11 for more details on bowel measurements.
- Various artefacts may be visible, ranging from foreign objects inserted into the rectum, vagina or urethra to surgical clips or brachytherapy seeds used to treat prostate cancer.

CHAPTER SUMMARY

- The pelvis and hips are inextricably linked, and whether pelvis imaging is obtained for femoral neck fractures or pelvic injuries, it is essential that the whole image is assessed.
- The pelvis is a ring bone, and an abnormality in one part may lead to a further abnormality within the ring, which could be another fracture or widening of the symphysis pubis or sacroiliac joints.
- Femoral neck fractures are classified as intracapsular and extracapsular, and there is a high incidence of osteonecrosis in intracapsular fractures.
- Surgical metalwork may show signs of loosening, periprosthetic fracture, infection or dislocation.
- There may be a subchondral lucency at the femoral head indicating osteonecrosis caused by previous trauma or Perthes disease in a child.
- Acetabular fractures are identified by assessing the six lines of Judet.
- Checking the sacral arcuate lines will help to identify sacral fractures.
- Dislocations in children are usually limited to younger children with DDH or CDH.
- A SUFE can be acute or chronic, and a lateral projection will show it in the early stages due to the posterior movement of the femoral epiphysis.
- Irritable hip may be apparent on an X-ray image if the gluteal fat stripes are bulging.
- Various soft tissue calcifications may be visible.
- The apophyses can avulse and appear as fragments in the soft tissues.

SECTION 4
AXIAL TRAUMA

11. SPINE

The spine is divided into the cervical, thoracic, lumbar, sacral and coccygeal sections. The focus of evaluation is assessing the integrity of three columns that run vertically through most of the spine (**Figure 11.1**). The columns are:

- the **anterior column** – the anterior part of the vertebral body and intervertebral disc; the anterior longitudinal ligament;
- the **middle column** – the posterior part of the vertebral body and intervertebral disc; the posterior longitudinal ligament;
- the **posterior column** – the posterior elements of the vertebral body (pedicles, laminae and spinous processes) and associated ligaments.

Spinal injuries can be classified according to the number of columns affected. An injury involving two or more of the columns is unstable.

Spinal injuries in children are relatively rare; however, when they do occur, they are usually within the cervical spine.

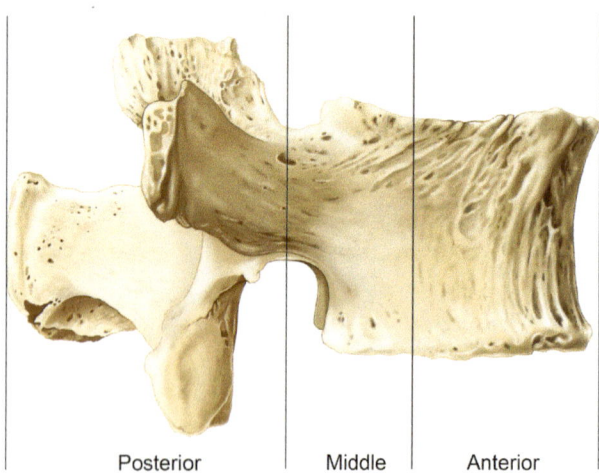

Posterior   Middle   Anterior

Figure 11.1 The three columns of the spine.

The most important function of the spine is to protect the spinal cord, which could be damaged in spinal trauma, with catastrophic results. In the phenomenon of spinal cord injury without radiographic abnormality (**SCIWORA**), the patient presents with symptoms of cord injury, but X-ray images and computed tomography (CT) scans do not identify an abnormality. The cervical spine is the most flexible of the three sections and is most affected, particularly in children, as their large head-to-body ratio and weakness in the neck muscles and ligaments results in significant movement of the cervical vertebrae, leading to cord damage without any visible abnormality.

Mechanisms of injury include hyperflexion, hyperextension, rotation, shearing and vertical compression/axial loading, and these commonly occur in road traffic collisions, sporting accidents or falls. There may also be any combination of these mechanisms, for example hyperflexion with axial loading or hyperextension with rotation. The resulting injury pattern can include compression or distraction fractures or translational injuries (the latter is a combination of a fracture with displacement of one vertebral body in relation to the adjacent vertebral body).

Hyperflexion is the most common mechanism of injury, such as that sustained during sudden deceleration in a road traffic collision, with injuries associated with anterior vertebral body compression or wedging often seen in the lower cervical spine or thoracolumbar junction. **Hyperextension** injuries are less common. Both mechanisms are often associated with a distraction injury in which there is abnormal widening within one of the spinal columns. For example, there may be increased widening of the anterior intervertebral disc space in a hyperextension injury, signifying anterior longitudinal ligament rupture.

Vertical compression or axial loading type injuries occur when excessive force is applied through a straight spine. Unlike a hyperflexion compression fracture, which occurs with the spine bent, the vertical compression injury results in the vertebral body being crushed and it is referred to as a **burst** fracture. This is a significant injury, as fracture fragments encroach into the spinal canal.

Rotational injuries cause one vertebral body to rotate in relation to the adjacent vertebral body. **Shearing** injuries result in one vertebral body moving in relation to the adjacent vertebral body. These two mechanisms may occur together and can result in significant fracture dislocation injuries.

While most spinal injuries are caused by indirect mechanisms as described above, direct force, such as that sustained during an assault, can also lead to spinal injuries. Abnormalities associated with common mechanisms of injury are found in **Table 11.1**. This is not an exhaustive list, but offers the more typical abnormalities associated with the mechanism of injury. Building on the ABCs method of evaluation, as introduced in Chapter 1, and assuming that adequacy has been checked, **Table 11.2** includes the more specific checks related to evaluation of the spine in general, and these will be built on throughout this chapter. Normal spine images summarising these additional checks for spine images are demonstrated in **Figure 11.2** for the cervical spine, in **Figure 11.3** for the thoracic spine and in **Figure 11.4** for the lumbar spine.

Table 11.1 Common mechanisms of injury and associated abnormalities in the spine.

Mechanism	Typical abnormality
Hyperflexion	Fracture involving the anterior vertebral body (flexion teardrop fracture)
	Spinous process fracture
	Reduction in the intervertebral disc space
	Malalignment of the vertebral bodies
	Splaying of the spinous processes
	Soft tissue swelling
Hyperextension	Widening of the anterior intervertebral disc space
	Malalignment of the vertebral bodies
	Avulsion fracture from the anteroinferior vertebral body (hyperextension teardrop fracture)
	Compression of the posterior vertebral body
	Fracture involving the posterior elements
	Soft tissue swelling
Vertical compression/ axial loading	Compression fracture of the vertebral body
Rotation	Malalignment of the vertebral bodies
	Loss of alignment at the facet joints
Shearing	Malalignment of the vertebral bodies
Direct impact	Spinous process fracture

Table 11.2 Summary of systematic checks to be made when evaluating the spine.

Focus	Points to consider
Bones	The anterior and posterior vertebral body heights should be similar. Reduction in the anterior body height may indicate a wedge fracture.
	The pedicles should be seen on the AP image in the thoracic and lumbar spine. If there is absence of a pedicle, this could indicate a metastatic lesion.
	Spinous processes must be identified on the AP image. A distraction fracture can result in one being 'missing'. The spinous processes on the lateral cervical spine should be convergent; that is, they should all be directed to a central point. Divergence of two spinous processes will indicate ligamentous injury.
	Check the remaining bony details of the visualised skeleton such as the pelvis and ribs.
Cartilaginous areas	The four lines of alignment on the lateral images are useful in assessing vertebral body alignment (see Figure 11.12).
	The intervertebral disc spaces should be equal throughout the spine and visible on both AP and lateral images.
	Assessment of the spinous processes, projected through the vertebral bodies on the AP image, is a good guide to alignment. Malalignment may indicate a rotational injury involving the facets.
	Facet joints should be assessed on the lateral image, with the superior facet of the lower vertebra being aligned with the inferior facet of the upper vertebra.
	The odontoid peg should be positioned centrally within C1 on the AP odontoid peg image, and the lateral masses of C1 and C2 should be aligned.
	The space between the odontoid peg and the anterior arch of C1 should be no more than 3 mm in an adult and 5 mm in a child (predental space).
	Check the sacroiliac joints on the AP lumbar spine.
Soft tissues	The prevertebral soft tissues should measure less than one-third of the vertebral body width at C1–C4 and no greater than the vertebral body width below C4. If there is an increase in the soft tissues, this could indicate a fracture or an infection.
	Check visible lung fields and abdomen.
	Check psoas shadow, if visible, for any deviation.
	Check the paraspinal line on the AP thoracic spine image.
	Calcification associated with the thyroid, hyoid, cricoid, tracheal and arytenoid cartilages may be seen.

AP, anteroposterior.

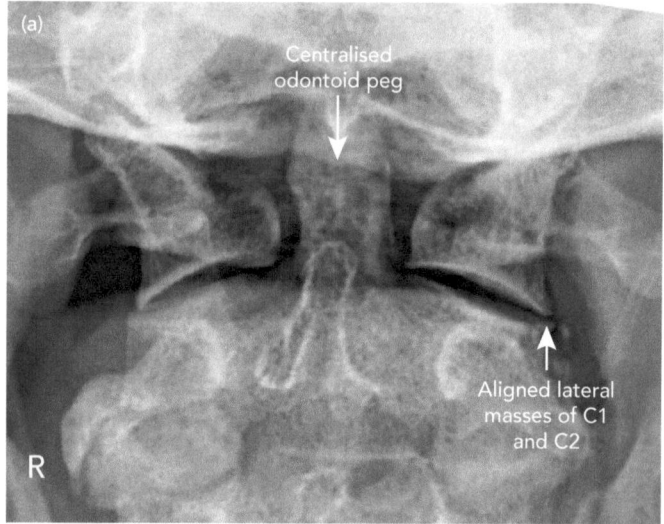

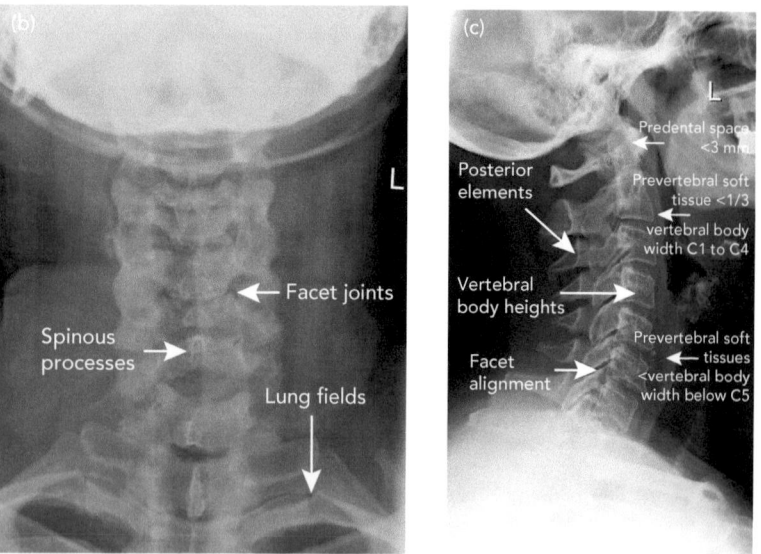

Figure 11.2 (a) Odontoid peg, (b) anteroposterior and (c) lateral cervical spine images demonstrating the checks that are unique to this area.

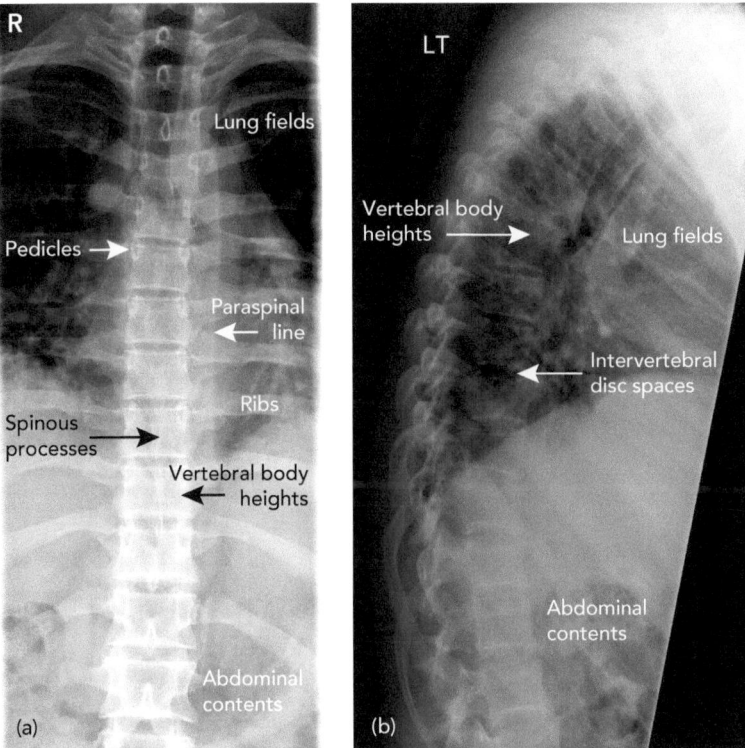

Figure 11.3 (a) Anteroposterior and (b) lateral thoracic spine images demonstrating the checks that are unique to this area.

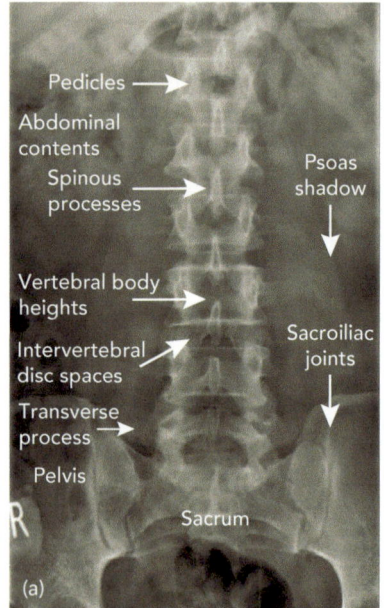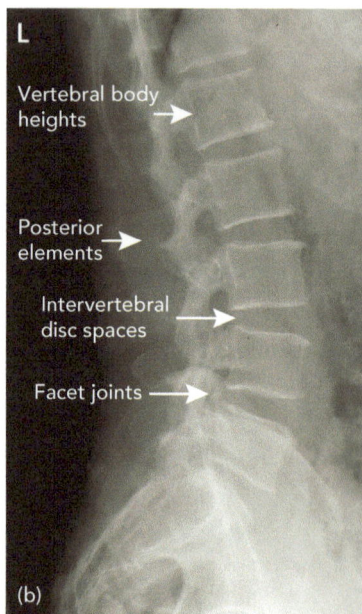

Figure 11.4 (a) Anteroposterior and (b) lateral lumbar spine images demonstrating the checks that are unique to this area.

When counting the lumbar vertebrae on the lateral image, there may appear to be six vertebrae. This is caused by lumbarisation of S1. The first sacral vertebra does not fuse with the remainder of the sacrum (see Figure 11.5a).

BONES

- Assess the vertebral bodies to ensure that there are no breaches in the cortex or areas of sclerosis that may indicate end-plate compressions. A beak-like appearance may also be seen on the anterosuperior margin in cases of superior end-plate compression.
- The anterior and posterior parts of the vertebral bodies should be approximately the same height. Reduction in the height of the anterior vertebral body may indicate a wedge fracture caused by a

hyperflexion injury and is often seen in patients with osteoporosis (**Figure 11.5a**). A reduction in the height of a vertebral body on the anteroposterior (AP) image may support this diagnosis (**Figure 11.5b**). In the thoracic spine, the anterior vertebral body height should be no less than 2 mm of the height of the posterior vertebral body, except at T11 and T12, which may demonstrate a slight physiological wedging.

■ Osteoporotic wedge fractures are commonly seen in older patients. Differentiation between a chronic and an acute fracture can be difficult in the absence of previous imaging for comparison. An acute fracture may have a buckle or a lucency and may be an isolated vertebral body fracture. A chronic fracture generally has increased sclerosis and there may be multiple contiguous vertebral body fractures.

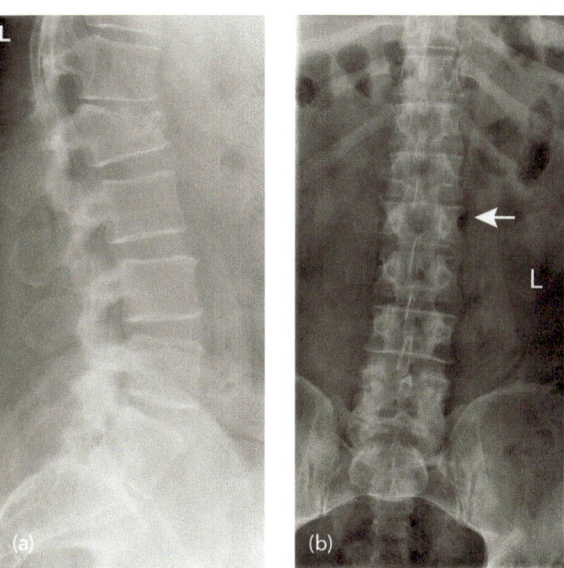

Figure 11.5 (a) Acute wedge fracture of L2 seen on a lateral lumbar spine image in which there is also lumbarisation of S1. (b) Reduction in height of L2 on the AP image.

> **Comment: wedge fracture of L2.**

- A flexion injury to the cervical spine is more likely to have a resultant abnormality between C4 and C7. This may be in the anteroinferior vertebral body, referred to as a **flexion teardrop fracture (Figure 11.6)**, and may be only a small triangular fragment. It is a significant injury due to damage to the anterior longitudinal ligament. With increasing severity of the flexion injury, the fracture can extend through the vertebral body resulting in damage to the posterior longitudinal ligament and posterior displacement of the vertebral body. Hyperflexion injuries can also result in a vertebral body compression or an anterior wedge fracture.
- A patient who has sustained a hyperflexion injury involving the torso, such as that which may be associated with wearing only a lap seat belt, is likely to have an injury in the thoracolumbar region involving a horizontal fracture through the spinous process, pedicles and posterior aspect of the vertebral body, referred to as a **Chance fracture**.

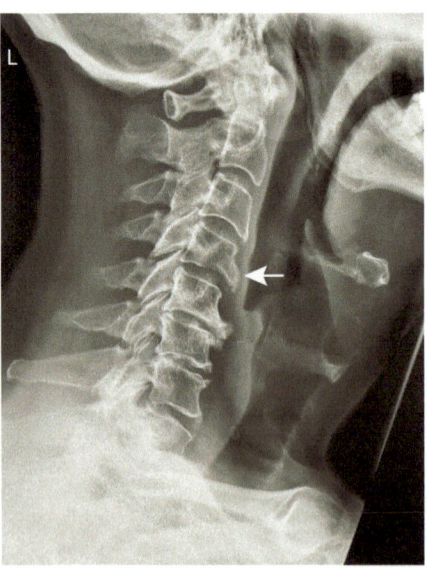

Figure 11.6 Lateral cervical spine image demonstrating a fracture through the anteroinferior margin of C4.

- Hyperextension injuries may cause compression in the posterior column resulting in fractures of the posterior elements (**Figure 11.7a**) and tension to the anterior longitudinal ligament leading to an avulsion fracture from the anteroinferior vertebral body margin (**Figure 11.7b**). This **extension teardrop fracture** is less severe than the flexion teardrop fracture. Hyperextension may also result in a fracture at the junction of the pedicles and laminae of C2 and subluxation of C2 in relation to C3, commonly known as the **Hangman's fracture (Figure 11.8)**.

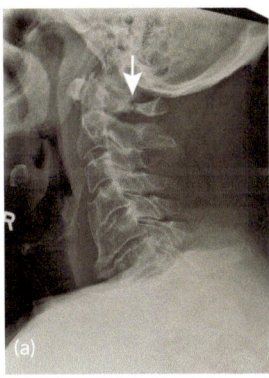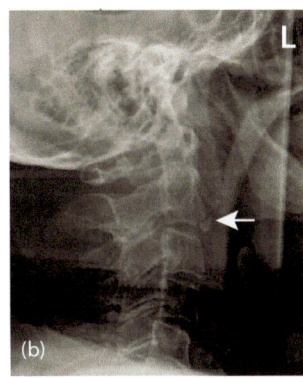

Figure 11.7 Lateral cervical spine images demonstrating (a) a fracture of the posterior arch of C1 and (b) an extension teardrop fracture of C2.

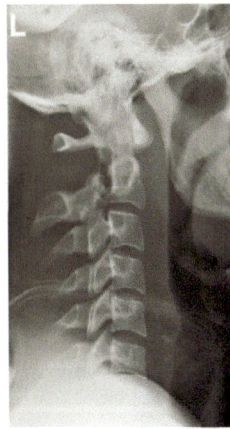

Figure 11.8 Lateral cervical spine image demonstrating a fracture through the posterior elements of C2.

165

- A **limbus vertebra** is a normal variant on lateral images of the cervical and lumbar spine, and occasionally in the thoracic spine, which may mimic a teardrop fracture. This is a result of the nucleus pulposus herniating through the ring apophysis. This is seen at the inferior corner of the vertebral body in the cervical spine (**Figure 11.9**) and the superior corner of the vertebral body in the lumbar spine.

- Fractures to the **odontoid peg** are often difficult to see on an X-ray image and can be caused by relatively insignificant trauma in older people, such as a fall from standing. Unfortunately, there is a high mortality rate in older people following an odontoid peg fracture.[1] On a normal lateral cervical spine image, there is an apparent ring, referred to as the **Harris ring**, created by the superimposition of C2 lateral masses onto the vertebral body (**Figure 11.10**). Identifying this ring will help in determining an odontoid peg fracture. If the ring is broken, then a fracture must be suspected.

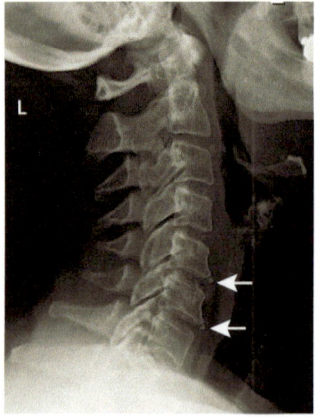

Figure 11.9 Lateral cervical spine image demonstrating limbus vertebrae at C5 and C6.

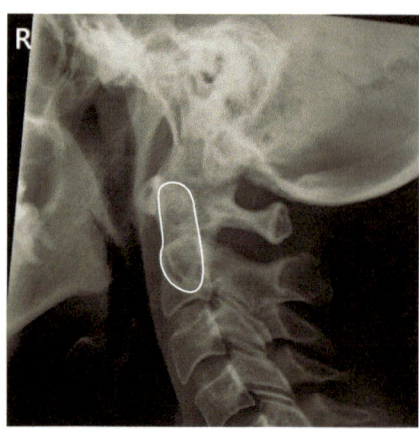

Figure 11.10 Lateral cervical spine image indicating the location of the Harris ring.

- The odontoid peg can fracture at its tip (type 1), its base (type 2) or below the base involving the vertebral body (type 3) (**Figure 11.11**). If the Harris ring is disrupted, this may indicate a type 2 or type 3 fracture, and other signs, such as soft tissue displacement, may be visible.

■ It is important not to mistake air within the oropharynx or the vertically orientated incisor line for a fracture of the odontoid peg (see Figure 1.1a).

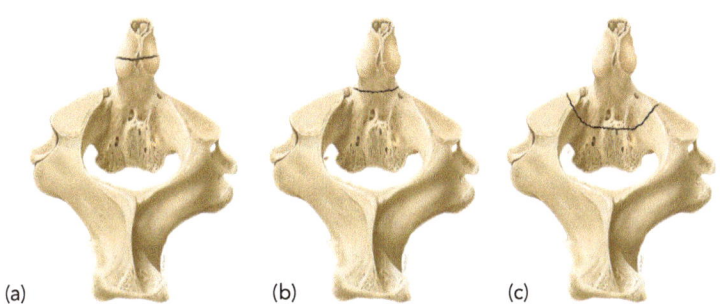

Figure 11.11 Odontoid peg fracture classification: (a) fracture at the tip (type 1), (b) fracture at the base (type 2) and (c) fracture below the base involving the vertebral body (type 3).

■ Assess the posterior elements. These are difficult to see on the lateral thoracic spine image but can be seen on the cervical and lumbar spine images. Direct impact may result in a fracture of the posterior elements, but they also occur following a hyperflexion or hyperextension injury. An isolated fracture of a spinous process in the cervical spine may be caused by excessive forces and twisting in the upper back and is often referred to as a **clay-shoveler fracture** when it is the lower cervical spine.

■ The pedicles should be seen clearly on the AP image (see Figures 11.3a and 11.4a). If there is absence of a pedicle, this could indicate a metastatic lesion.

■ Transverse processes must be assessed where they can be seen. In particular, the transverse processes of L5 may be fractured in a significant pelvic injury and may be the only radiological sign of an unstable pelvis.

CARTILAGINOUS AREAS

- Alignment, indicating that the intervertebral joints (intervertebral disc space and facet joints) are intact, is assessed using four spinal lines (**Figure 11.12**):

    1. **anterior spinal line** – the anterior borders of the vertebral bodies and the location of the anterior longitudinal ligament;
    2. **posterior spinal line** – the posterior borders of the vertebral bodies and the location of the posterior longitudinal ligament; the normal paediatric cervical spine may demonstrate some disruption in this line as a normal variant (**Figure 11.13**);
    3. **spinolaminar line** – the junction of the lamina and spinous processes;
    4. **spinous process tips** – the length of these can be variable, so this line does not have much value in identifying abnormality.

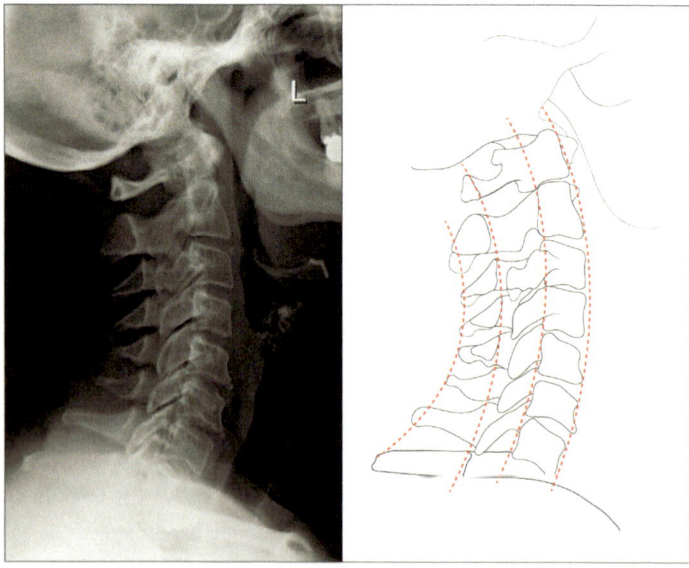

Figure 11.12 Lines of alignment demonstrated on a lateral cervical spine image.

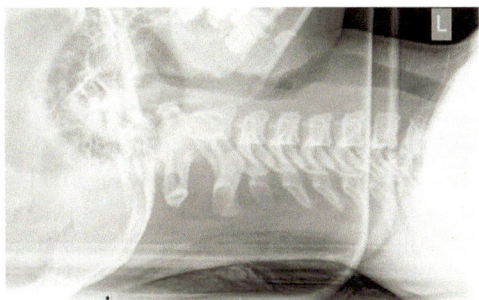

Figure 11.13 Lateral cervical spine image demonstrating a physiological pseudosubluxation at C2/3 in a child.

- Malalignment may be apparent, a condition referred to as **spondylolisthesis**. **Anterolisthesis** is anterior slip in relation to the adjacent vertebra (**Figure 11.14a**) and **retrolisthesis** is a posterior slip (**Figure 11.14b**). Both can be caused by trauma or degeneration and may be an incidental finding. They are graded from grade 1 (less than 25% slip) to grade 3 (greater than 50% slip). **Retropulsion** is the term used if there are fracture fragments seen to have moved posteriorly into the spinal canal.

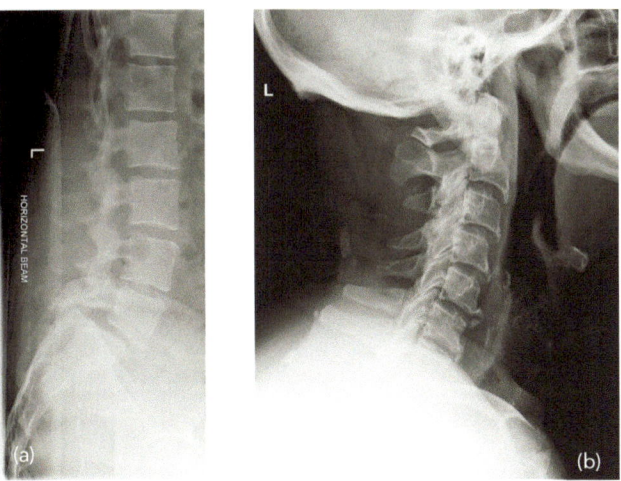

Figure 11.14 (a) Lateral lumbar spine image demonstrating anterolisthesis at L5/S1. (b) Lateral cervical spine image demonstrating retrolisthesis of C4.

- The vertebral bodies should be normally aligned on the AP image. This is assessed on the AP cervical spine image by checking the undulation of the vertebral bodies laterally for any sudden change. A flexion injury, with axial compression and rotation or shearing, will lead to lateral displacement of the vertebral body.

- On the odontoid peg image, the lateral masses of C1 may overhang the lateral masses of C2 by up to 6 mm in a child under the age of 4 years. In all other patients, the odontoid peg should be positioned centrally within C1, and the lateral masses should be aligned (Figure 11.2a). An offset of the lateral masses of C1 and C2 greater than 7 mm indicates a fracture of C1 caused by axial loading; this is referred to as a **Jefferson** fracture (**Figure 11.15**).

- Increased distance between the lateral masses of C1 and C2 may also indicate a fracture of C1 and/or C2 (**Figure 11.16**).

- The normal distance of the predental space as seen on the lateral image is less than 3 mm in an adult and less than 4 mm in a child (Figure 11.2c). Widening of this space is highly suspicious of a fracture of C1 or of the odontoid peg.

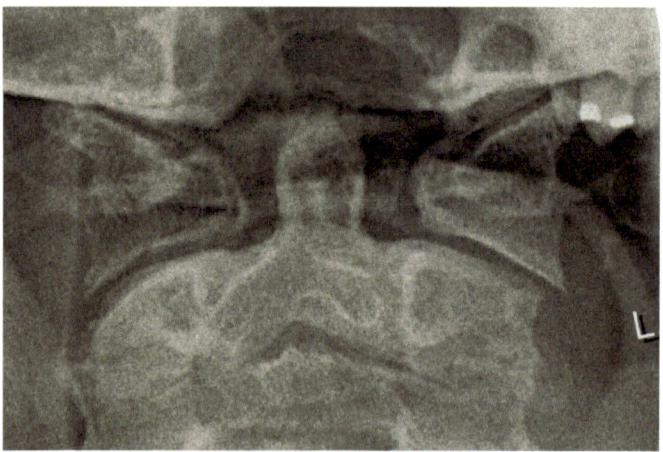

Figure 11.15 Odontoid peg image demonstrating widening between the odontoid peg and left lateral mass of C1 and the overhang of this lateral mass in relation to the lateral mass of C2.

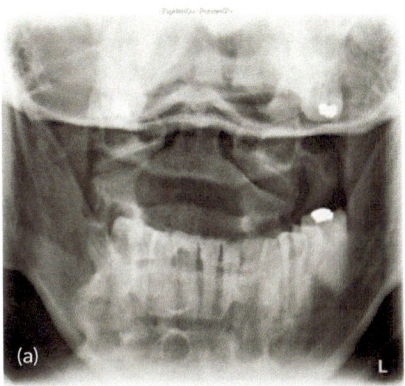 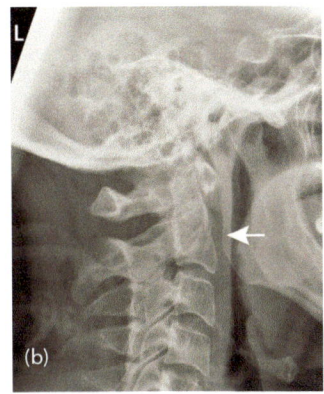

Figure 11.16 Fracture of the odontoid peg demonstrated by (a) an increased distance between the left lateral masses of C1 and C2 on the odontoid peg image and (b) irregularity in the anterior cortex of C1 on the cropped lateral cervical spine image.

■ Facet joint injuries can occur following a flexion-distraction injury. On the lateral image, the superior facet of the lower vertebra should be anterior to and aligned with the inferior facet of the upper vertebra (Figure 11.2c). Disruption to this appearance, often affecting the spinal lines, is highly suspicious of injury, either a subluxation in which there is still some contact between the upper and lower articular surfaces of the facet joint (**perched facets**) or a dislocation in which the lower articular surface moves behind the upper articular surface (**locked facets**) (**Figure 11.17**). This can be unilateral or bilateral and will manifest as malalignment with anterior slip of the vertebral body. It will also be evident on the AP image with widening of the affected facet joint or the uncovertebral joint in the cervical spine (**Figure 11.18**). Unilateral facet dislocation, sometimes referred to as rotary subluxation of the vertebral body, is indicated if the amount of anterior slip is less than 25% of the vertebral body width. Bilateral facet dislocation is indicated if the slip is greater than 25%.

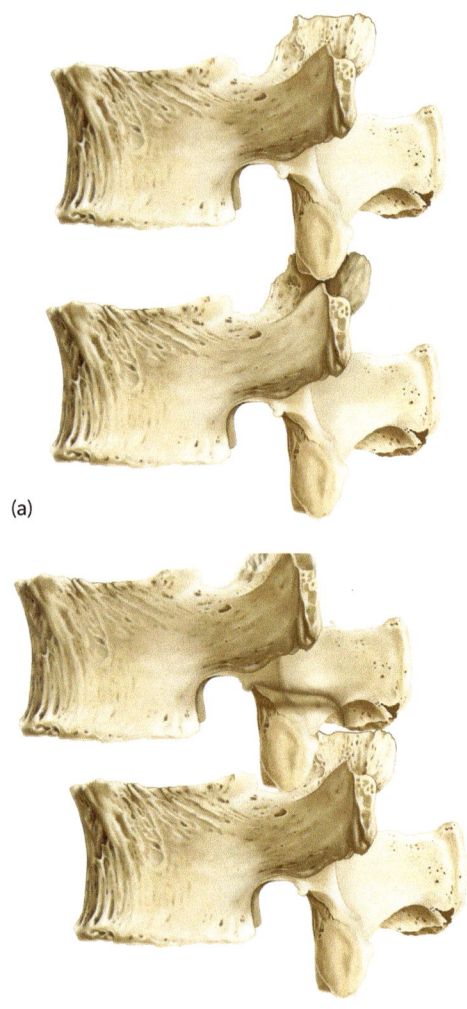

(a)

(b)

Figure 11.17 Diagram illustrating (a) perched facets and (b) locked facets.

- There may be slight malalignment in the degenerative spine, but there will be associated degenerative changes and no history of trauma (see Figure 11.25).

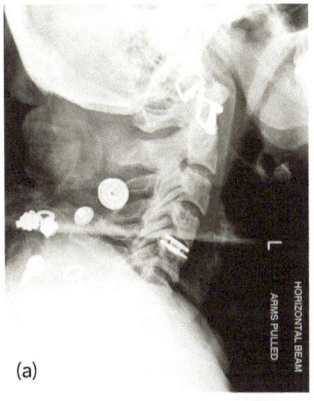

(a)

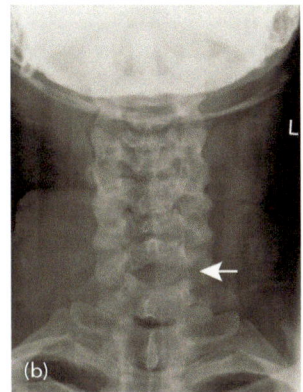

(b)

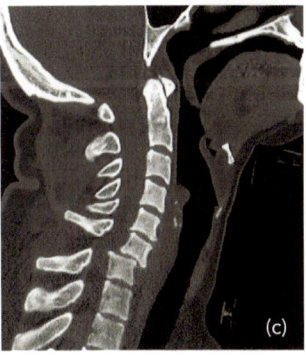

(c)

Figure 11.18 (a) Lateral cervical spine image with inadequate visualisation of the cervicothoracic junction. (b) AP cervical spine image demonstrating irregularity at the uncovertebral joints. (c) CT scan indicating facet dislocation at C6/7.

Comment: on X-ray images – widening of C6/7 left uncovertebral joint and splaying of the spinous processes indicate significant injury at C6/7.

- The spinous processes must be checked on the AP image. They should be aligned with each other and the difference in distance between adjacent spinous processes should be minimal. Increase in the distance or malalignment of a spinous process may support an appearance on the lateral image of posterior ligament disruption with or without vertebral body displacement. Note the increased distance between the spinous processes of C6 and C7 on both the AP and the lateral images in Figure 11.18.

- The normal lordotic appearance of the cervical and lumbar spines may be lost, but if the vertebral bodies remain normally aligned, then this generally indicates muscle spasm. If the long axis of adjacent spinous processes is divergent, there may be posterior ligament disruption (**Figure 11.19**).

- Although not true malalignment of the vertebral bodies, some patients may have an abnormal lateral curve of the spine (**scoliosis**) or an exaggerated anterior curve in the upper thoracic spine (**kyphosis**). Idiopathic scoliosis is a disease for which there is no known cause and is generally diagnosed in children or adolescents. A scoliosis can be one or more lateral curves of the spine (**Figure 11.20**). The whole spine needs to be included on imaging so that measurements can be made to assess the degree of curvature. The vertebral bodies must also be clearly seen, as known causes of scoliosis include a development abnormality of the vertebra or a benign tumour (osteoid osteoma), which causes muscle spasms resulting in scoliosis.

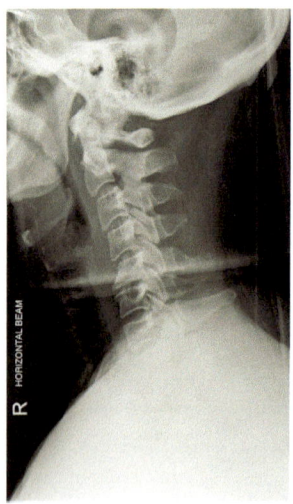

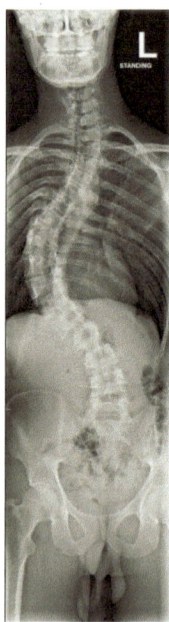

Figure 11.19 Lateral cervical spine image demonstrating loss of lordosis and splaying of C4/5 indicating ligamentous injury.

Figure 11.20 AP whole spine image demonstrating idiopathic double scoliosis.

SOFT TISSUES

- The prevertebral soft tissues (**retropharyngeal space**) should measure less than one-third of the vertebral body width at C1–C4 and no greater than the vertebral body width below C4 (Figure 11.2c). If there is an increase in the soft tissues, this could indicate a fracture or an infection (**Figure 11.21**).

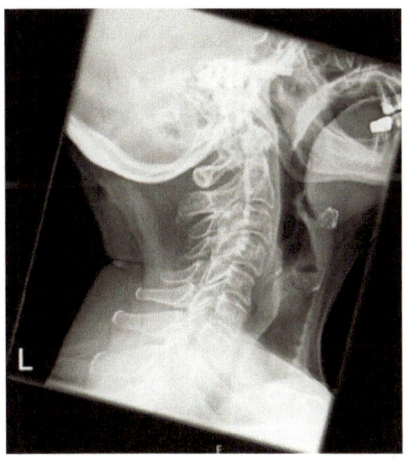

Figure 11.21 Lateral cervical spine image demonstrating increased prevertebral soft tissue swelling anterior to C5.

- On the AP thoracic spine image, the **paraspinal line** may be visible on the left side. This is created by the boundary between the left lung and the posterior mediastinum and sits in close proximity to the spine (**Figure 11.22**). Deviation may indicate underlying pathology such as infection or haematoma from a fracture.
- The visualised lung fields must be evaluated. These may demonstrate known disease that does not need any further action. However, in some cases, it will be necessary to expedite an urgent report or inform the referring clinician if immediate medical attention is needed. If a lesion is identified, it is not the role of the practitioner evaluating the images to determine if it is benign or

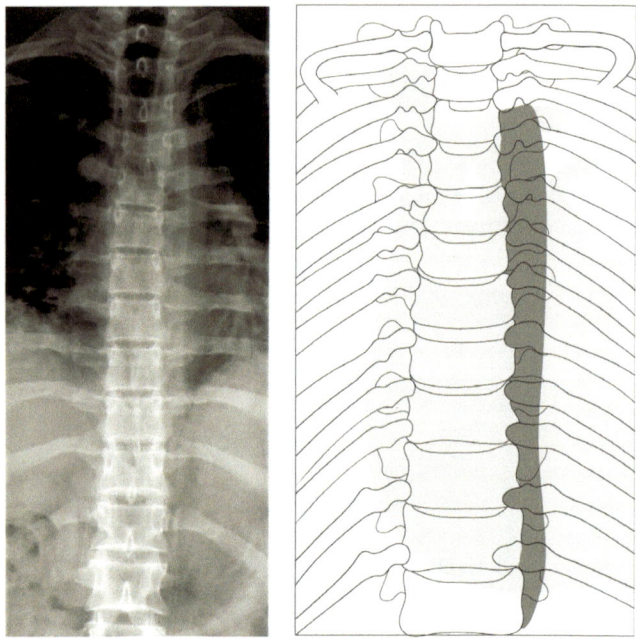

Figure 11.22 AP thoracic spine demonstrating the position of the paraspinal line.

aggressive, but it is their responsibility to highlight the finding and expedite a formal report by bringing it to the attention of a reporting practitioner. Further detail is given in Chapter 6 on possible lung pathologies that may be seen.

■ The abdomen must be assessed if included on images. Numerous features indicating abdominal pathology may be seen. These should be brought to the attention of a reporting practitioner or the referring clinician.

– The psoas shadow is not always visible, but, where it is, it is seen bilaterally extending from L1 to the iliac crest (Figure 11.4a). Disruption, such as loss of the shadow on one side of the spine or a bulging line, may be a sign of pathology such as a spinal tumour or abscess.

– Vascular calcification, due to **atherosclerosis**, may be present and is commonly seen on the lateral lumbar spine image. Widening within the aorta may indicate an aortic aneurysm (**Figure 11.23**), which can be a cause of back pain. While not diagnostic of abdominal aortic aneurysm, it may raise concerns and prompt further investigations.

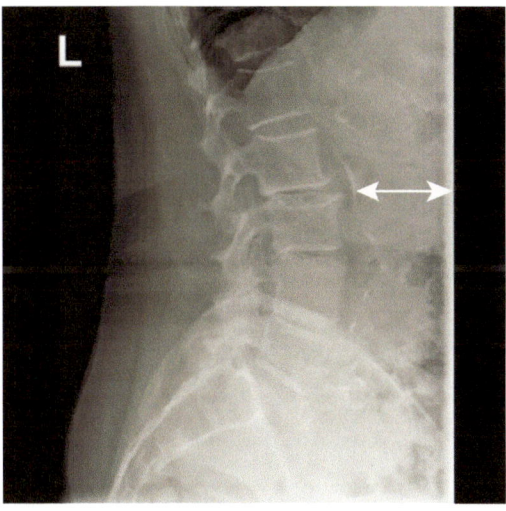

Figure 11.23 Lateral lumbar spine images demonstrating aortic calcification with widening of the aorta.

– Signs of **bowel obstruction** may be visible on the AP lumbar spine image. The normal diameter of the bowel is:

   o less than 3 cm in the small bowel;
   o less than 6 cm in the large bowel;
   o less than 9 cm in the caecum.

   The bowel is dilated if the measurements are greater than this and obstruction must be considered (**Figure 11.24**).

– Renal stones may be visible within the kidneys or ureters.
– Gallstones may be visible within the gallbladder or biliary tree.

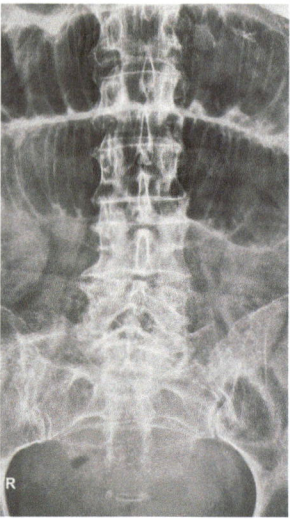

Figure 11.24 AP lumbar spine image demonstrating an increased diameter of the small bowel indicating small bowel obstruction.

- A normal variant that may be seen in the posterior aspect of the cervical spine is calcification of the **nuchal ligament (Figure 11.25)**.
- Calcification of the cricoid, hyoid, thyroid, tracheal or arytenoid cartilages may be seen in the anterior soft tissues (Figure 11.25).
- Lateral cervical spine images are often obtained to identify possible foreign bodies, either inhaled or ingested. Metallic foreign bodies are easy to see, but fish bones are the most commonly ingested foreign bodies and these are not always radiopaque. Loss of the normal cervical lordosis can be associated with impaction of a foreign body and there may also be soft tissue swelling at the level of impaction **(Figure 11.26)**.

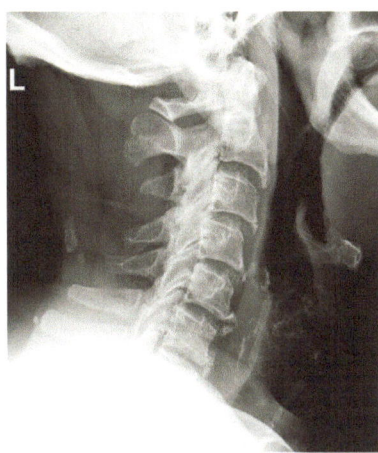

Figure 11.25 Lateral cervical spine image demonstrating densities in the soft tissues posterior to the spine in keeping with nuchal ligament calcification, and densities in the soft tissues anterior to the spine in keeping with calcification of the tracheal cartilages and hyoid.

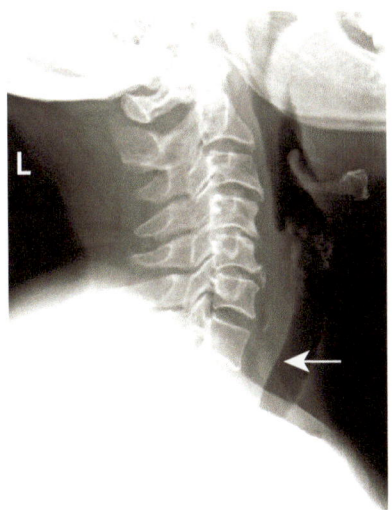

Figure 11.26 Lateral cervical spine image demonstrating a retained foreign body with soft tissue swelling.

Comment: **foreign body anterior to C7.**

CHAPTER SUMMARY

- The focus of evaluation is assessing the integrity of three columns. An injury involving two or more of the columns is unstable.
- SCIWORA is a phenomenon in which the spinal cord is injured but a radiographic abnormality is not identified.
- The anterior and posterior vertebral body heights should be approximately the same height.
- There are many different types of fractures and careful evaluation is required to identify the often-subtle appearances.
- A limbus vertebra is a normal variant that can mimic a teardrop fracture.
- An odontoid peg fracture can be difficult to identify. The Harris ring can be useful in assessing the odontoid peg.
- Vertebral body alignment is assessed using four spinal lines.
- Facet joint injuries can result in perched or locked facets.
- The normal predental space distance is 3 mm in an adult and 4 mm in a child.
- The prevertebral soft tissues should measure less than one-third of the vertebral body width at C1–C4 and no greater than the vertebral body width below C4. If there is an increase in the soft tissues, this could indicate a fracture or an infection.
- On the AP thoracic spine image, the paraspinal line may be deviated, indicating underlying pathology such as infection or haematoma from a fracture.
- Signs of bowel obstruction may be visible on the AP lumbar spine image, with the normal diameter of the bowel being less than 3 cm in the small bowel, less than 6 cm in the large bowel and less than 9 cm in the caecum.

REFERENCE

1. Esseonu, K., Oduoza, U., Fakouri, B. and Liantis, P. Fractures of the odontoid peg of the cervical spine. *Injury* 2020;51(11):2429–2436.

12. FACIAL BONES

Skull and facial bone injuries occur following direct low- or high-impact trauma (**Table 12.1**). Skull X-ray images have largely been superseded by computed tomography (CT) scans, but there is still a place for skull imaging in some instances, such as when performing skeletal surveys or on the rare occasion that CT scanning is unavailable. Skull fractures associated with suspected physical abuse will be discussed in Chapter 13. The focus of this chapter will be on evaluating images of the facial skeleton. The temporomandibular joints (TMJs) will be included, as they are often imaged alongside the mandible.

A patient who has sustained facial injuries is likely to present with facial lacerations, limited eye movements, malocclusion or visual disturbance. This is more common in the young adult male population, with very few facial bone fractures occurring in children. While projectional imaging may have been used to identify the presence of facial trauma, a CT scan will be required to determine the extent of any injury due to the complexity of the facial skeleton (**Figure 12.1**). The facial skeleton can be divided into the mandible and the upper face, which includes the maxilla, zygoma and orbits. The most common injuries involve the zygoma, an important bone in the physical appearance of a person, so correct identification of a fracture is essential in restoring the patient's facial features. Of all facial bone fractures, orbital floor blowout fractures are the most clinically and surgically significant, yet are often subtle on X-ray images.

Table 12.1 Common mechanisms of injury and associated abnormalities in the facial bones.

Mechanism	Typical abnormality
Direct impact (e.g. sporting injury or assault)	Orbital floor fracture Zygomatic arch fracture Nasal bone fracture
Fall, low impact	Zygoma fracture
Road traffic collision or high-impact trauma	Le Fort fractures (with or without head injury)

Frontal View

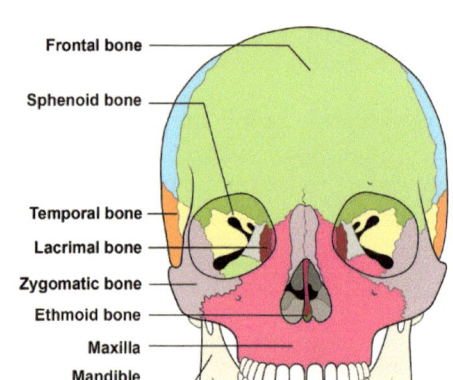

Frontal bone
Sphenoid bone
Temporal bone
Lacrimal bone
Zygomatic bone
Ethmoid bone
Maxilla
Mandible
Ramus
Body

(a)

Lateral View

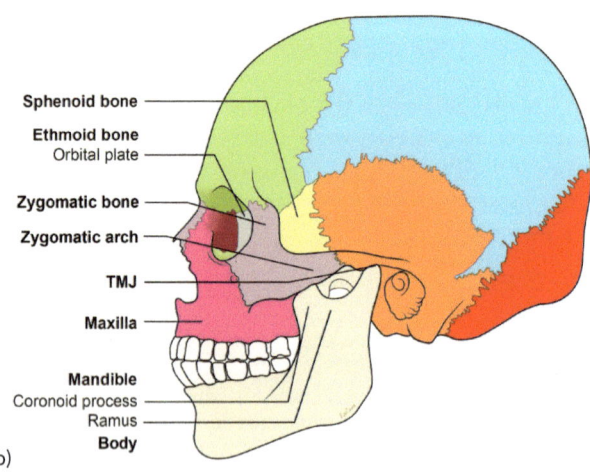

Sphenoid bone
Ethmoid bone
Orbital plate
Zygomatic bone
Zygomatic arch
TMJ
Maxilla
Mandible
Coronoid process
Ramus
Body

(b)

Figure 12.1 Anatomy of the skull and facial bones in (a) anteroposterior and (b) lateral views.

Numerous methods have been proposed for evaluating upper facial bone X-ray images, but there are two often used alongside each other to ensure that the whole of the facial anatomy has been assessed. The first is **Dolan's lines**, which have the appearance of an elephant, often referred to as Dolan's elephant (**Figure 12.2a**). The second is **McGrigor–Campbell lines (Figure 12.2b)**. Each has three virtual lines which should demonstrate symmetry. A lack of symmetry is likely to indicate an abnormality.

Building on the ABCs method of evaluation, as introduced in Chapter 1, and assuming that adequacy has been checked, **Table 12.2** includes the more specific checks related to evaluation of the facial skeleton, and these will be built on throughout this chapter. Normal images summarising these additional checks for facial skeleton images are demonstrated in **Figure 12.3** for upper facial bones and in **Figure 12.4** for the mandible.

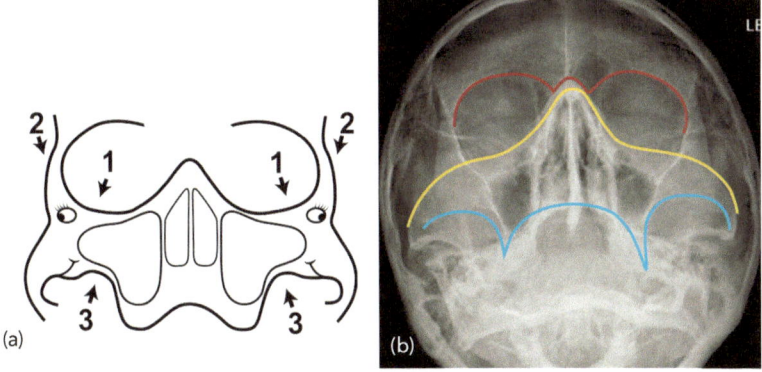

Figure 12.2 Lines of facial bone assessment: (a) Dolan's lines and (b) McGrigor–Campbell lines.

Facial Bones

Table 12.2 Summary of systematic checks to be made when evaluating the facial bones.

Focus	Points to consider
Bones	The nasal septum is normally straight and not deviated from the midline.
	Asymmetry of the face is often a useful indicator for a fracture. The zygoma should be assessed carefully, as fractures here are common. The margins, including the zygomatic arch and the lateral wall of the maxillary sinus, are the most vulnerable.
	Mandible fractures tend to be bilateral. A single fracture can occur, but a careful assessment should be undertaken for subtle second fractures or TMJ injury.
Cartilaginous areas	Cartilage is important in TMJ dysfunction. Both TMJs should align with the mandibular fossae.
	The frontozygomatic sutures should be equal bilaterally and without any widening.
	Alignment of the teeth is important in assessing the severity of a mandible fracture and in restoring function during fixation.
Soft tissues	Fluid levels in the maxillary sinus can be a sign of an underlying bony injury (not to be confused with thickening seen in sinusitis).
	The maxillary sinus should be clear of any soft tissue signs. The teardrop sign in the superior aspect of the maxillary sinus suggests an orbital floor 'blowout' fracture.
	The orbits should be assessed for reduced density tracking the superior aspect of the orbit, known as the 'black eyebrow' sign, which is another feature suggesting an orbital floor 'blowout' fracture or fracture involving the ethmoid sinuses.

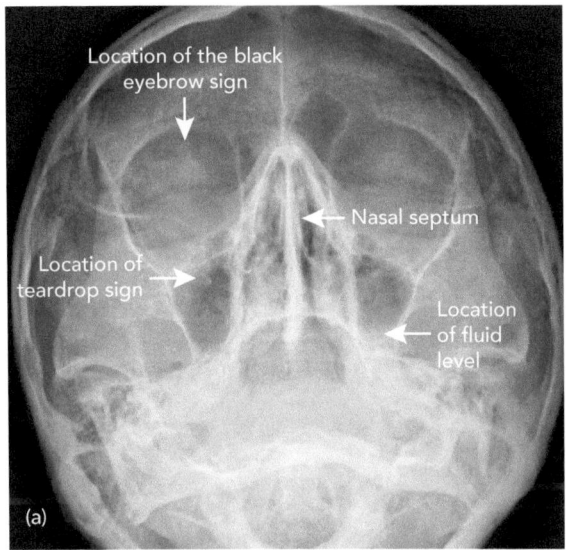

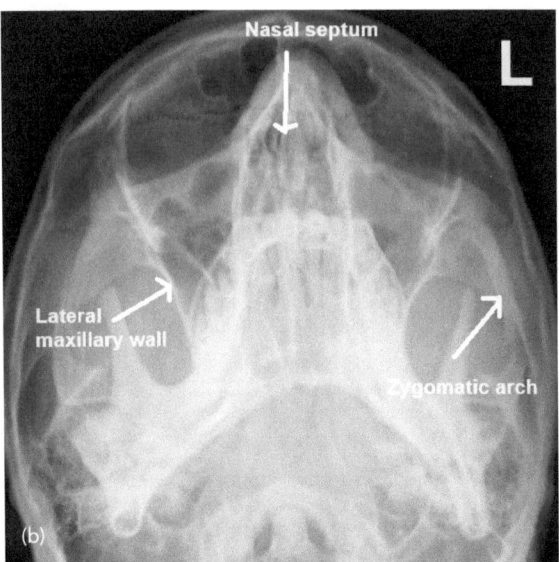

Figure 12.3 (a) Occipitomental image and (b) occipitomental 30° image of upper facial bones demonstrating the checks that are unique to this area.

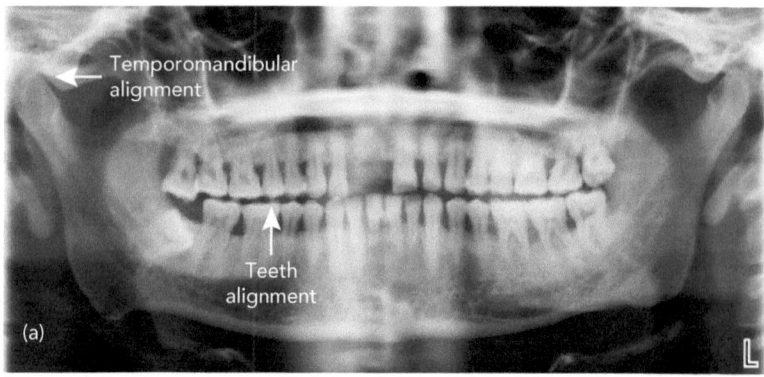

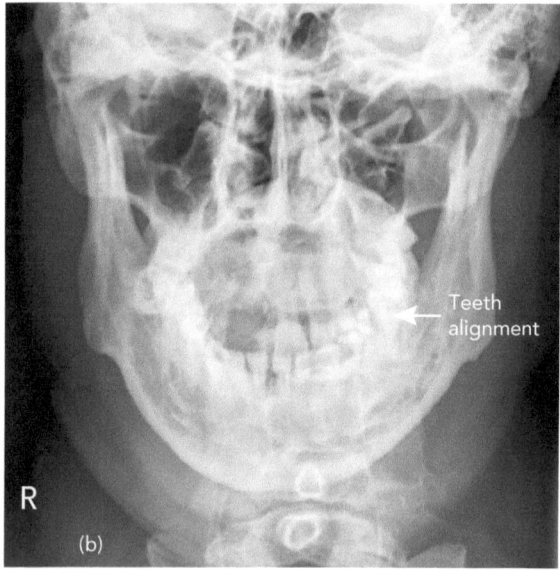

Figure 12.4 (a) Orthopantomogram and (b) posteroanterior mandible demonstrating normal anatomy.

BONES

- **Nasal bone** images are not routinely performed within the UK, but it may be possible to see nasal septum deviation on facial bone images, suggesting a nasal bone fracture. Clinical information is relevant, as it is not possible to differentiate between an acute and a chronic deviation.
- Facial symmetry can be assessed using Dolan's lines and/or McGrigor–Campbell lines, and asymmetry is a useful indicator of a fracture. The zygomatic arch and the lateral wall of the maxillary sinus are vulnerable to fracture from direct impact.
- The frontozygomatic suture may be widened and this may indicate a fracture involving the **zygomaticomaxillary complex (Figure 12.5)**.[1] This was previously called the tripod fracture, referring to the three elements of the injury, which result in the zygoma becoming isolated from the remaining facial bones:

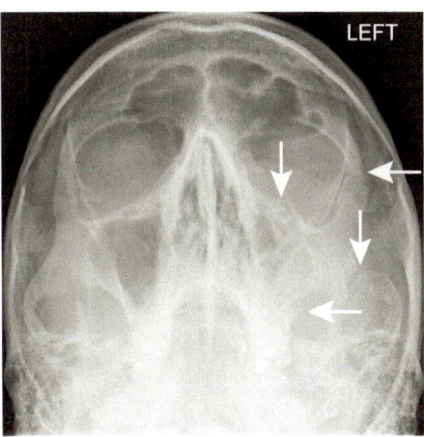

Figure 12.5 Occipitomental image of facial bones demonstrating a zygomaticomaxillary complex fracture.

Comment: fractures of the left zygomatic arch, left maxillary sinus lateral wall and left inferior orbital floor and widening of the left frontozygomatic suture.

1. fracture of the lateral orbital wall and/or widening of the frontozygomatic suture;
2. fracture of the zygomatic arch and/or widening of the temporozygomatic suture;
3. fracture of the zygoma at the inferior orbital floor and extending through the maxillary sinus with a fracture often seen in the lateral wall of the sinus; the zygomaticomaxillary suture may also be widened.

- Isolated **zygomatic arch** fractures can occur and may involve the zygomaticotemporal suture. There should be symmetry in the zygomatic arches, and abnormality should be suspected if one zygomatic arch appears different from the other (**Figure 12.6**).

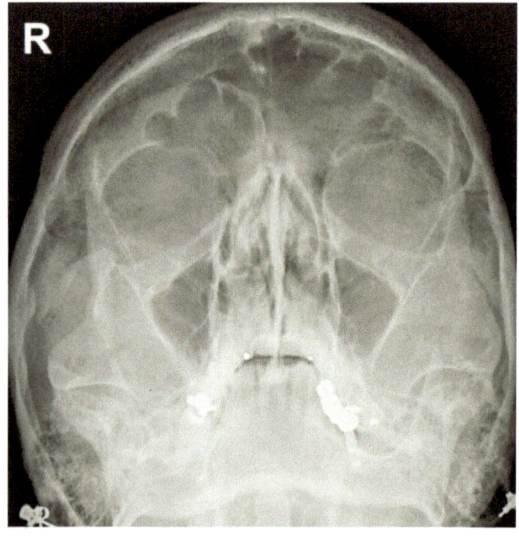

Figure 12.6 Occipitomental facial bones image demonstrating an isolated right zygomatic arch fracture.

- Facial bone fractures are often classified using the **Le Fort classification** method. This indicates the amount of separation of the midface from the skull base because of trauma.

  - Le Fort type 1 involves the maxilla: the fracture is transverse through the maxillary sinuses or the alveolar process, creating separation of the maxilla from the rest of the face.
  - Le Fort type 2 involves the zygomaticomaxillary suture, the inferior orbital floor and the nasal bones: it is pyramidal with the upper teeth at the base and the nasal bridge at the apex. This creates separation of the midface.
  - Le Fort type 3 involves the frontozygomatic sutures, the frontomaxillary sutures and the zygomatic arches: fracture extends through the medial and lateral walls of the orbits and results in separation of the whole face.

- **Mandible fractures** are common injuries associated with direct-impact trauma. The mandible is a ring bone equivalent, so careful assessment for a second injury is required (**Figure 12.7**). A second fracture may not be visible on the orthopantomogram (OPG), and a posteroanterior mandible image is essential in all cases of mandibular trauma.

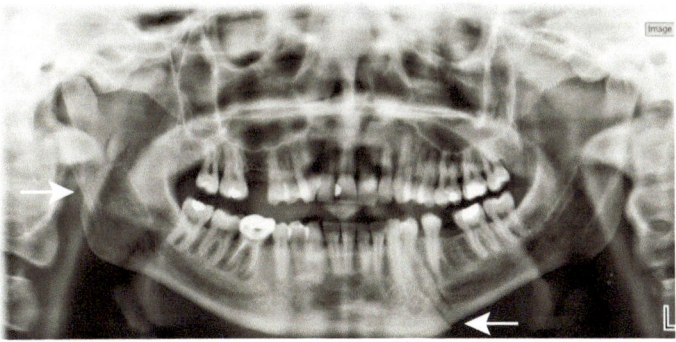

Figure 12.7 OPG image demonstrating two fractures in the mandible.

Comment: fractures through the left mandibular body and the right ramus.

- **Dentoalveolar fractures** involve the tooth-bearing region of either the mandible or the maxilla (**Figure 12.8**). Fractures in this region in the mandible are usually easy to identify; however, fractures involving the maxillary dentoalveolar region may be harder to see. Like bilateral fractures of the mandible, dentoalveolar fractures in the maxilla often lead to a mobile bony segment.

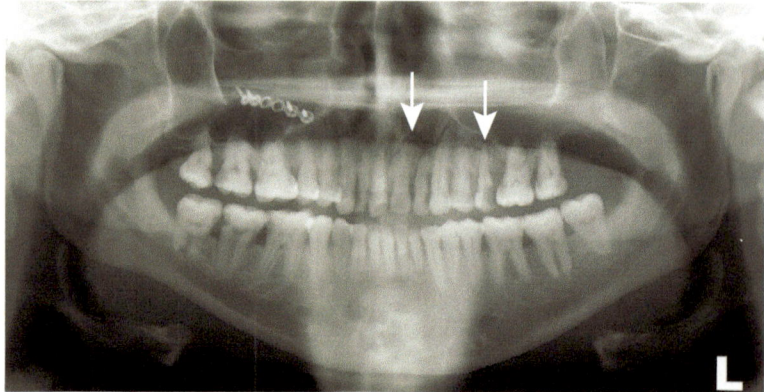

Figure 12.8 OPG image demonstrating a lucent line in the dentoalveolar region of the left maxilla indicating a fracture.

> Comment: **fracture through the dentoalveolar region of the left maxilla.**

CARTILAGINOUS AREAS

- The only cartilaginous area for consideration in facial bone anatomy is the **TMJ**, comprising the mandibular condyle, articular disc and mandibular fossa. Normal TMJ movement involves forward motion of the condyle from the fossa, known as translation. The normal full extent of translation is the articular tubercle (**Figure 12.9a**). Sometimes the articular disc can move forward slightly, causing reduced movement, locking, clicking or a feeling of subluxation or dislocation. A true dislocation of the TMJ occurs when the condyle moves anterior to the articular tubercle

(**Figure 12.9b**) and this is clinically obvious, as the mouth is in a fixed open position. The patient will be unable to close their mouth on the OPG bite block; the resulting characteristic image will show a large gap between the upper and lower teeth (**Figure 12.10**). The mandibular condyles will be positioned significantly anterior to the articular tubercles, more than in normal movement. TMJ dislocation is normally bilateral, although unilateral dislocation can occur.

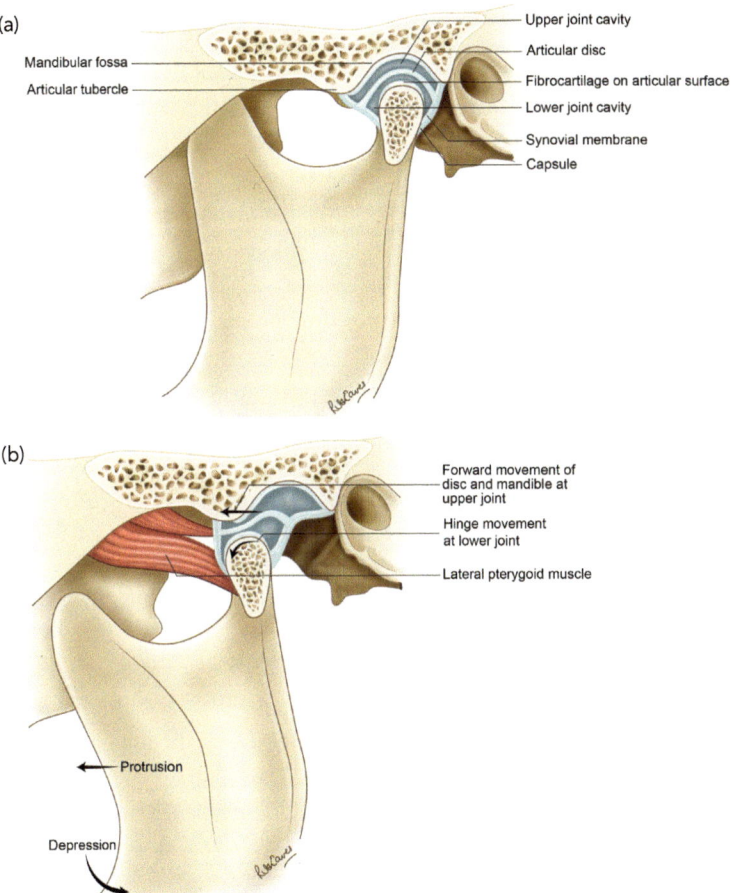

Figure 12.9 (a) Normal anatomy of the TMJ. (b) Forward movement of the mandible at the TMJ.

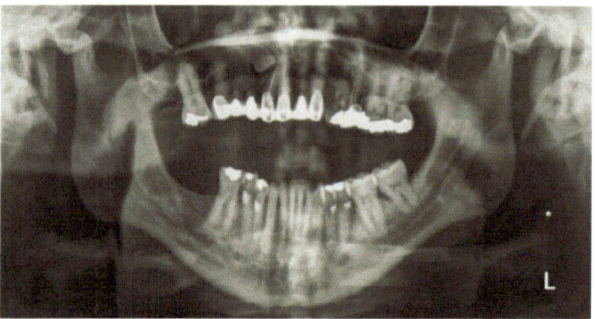

Figure 12.10 OPG image demonstrating bilateral TMJ dislocations.

> Comment: **bilateral dislocation of the TMJs; no fracture on this single view.**

SOFT TISSUES

- If a fracture involves the sinuses, air may track from the sinus and be seen in an unusual location on the images. This is most often seen when a fracture breaches the maxillary or ethmoid sinuses and air from within the sinus passes through the fracture and tracks around the orbit, visible as an area of radiolucency within the superior aspect of the orbit, referred to as a '**black eyebrow**' sign (**Figure 12.11**). If this is seen bilaterally, it is usually a normal variant.
- Opacification within the maxillary sinus can be one of the following.
    - First, it may be herniation of soft tissues through a blowout fracture in the orbital floor, if the soft tissue is seen in the upper aspect of the maxillary sinus, which is referred to as a '**teardrop**' sign (Figure 12.11). This is caused by direct trauma to the orbit in which there is a dramatic increase in ocular pressure. The fracture may not be visible, as the orbital margin is stronger than the orbital floor, so this

may appear intact. Maxillary sinus polyps have a similar appearance and careful consideration of the presenting clinical indication is advised.

- Second, it may be a sign of fracture if there is a horizontal **fluid level** indicating blood accumulation within the maxillary sinus (**Figure 12.12**).
- Finally, it may be sinus disease if there is no fluid level.

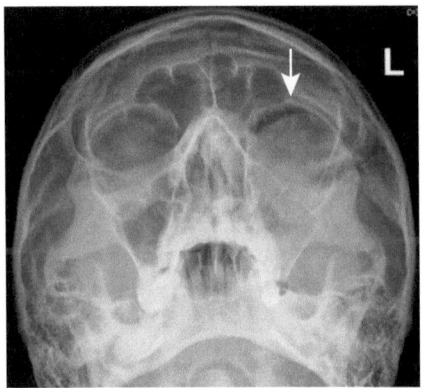

Figure 12.11 Occipitomental facial bones image demonstrating a left black eyebrow sign and a teardrop sign in the upper left maxillary sinus.

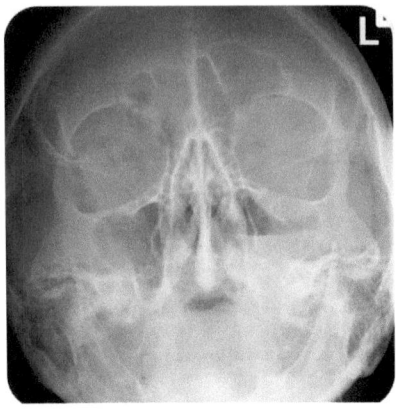

Figure 12.12 Occipitomental facial bones image demonstrating a fluid level in the left maxillary sinus indicating a fracture.

CHAPTER SUMMARY

- Skull X-ray images have largely been superseded by CT scans, but there is still a place for skull imaging in some instances, such as when performing skeletal surveys or on the rare occasion that CT scanning is unavailable.
- The most common facial bone injuries involve the zygoma.
- The most clinically and surgically significant facial bone injuries are orbital floor blowout fractures, but these are often subtle on X-ray images.
- Dolan's and McGrigor–Campbell lines are useful to ensure that the whole of the facial anatomy has been assessed and can help to identify a lack of symmetry, which may indicate injury.
- A zygomaticomaxillary complex injury results in the zygoma becoming isolated from the remaining facial bones.
- Le Fort classification indicates the amount of separation of the midface from the skull base because of trauma.
- Mandible fractures are common injuries associated with direct-impact trauma.
- A 'black eyebrow' sign occurs when a fracture involves the sinuses and air tracks from the sinus and around the orbit, visible as an area of radiolucency within the superior aspect of the orbit.
- A 'teardrop' sign is soft tissue in the upper aspect of the maxillary sinus caused by herniation of soft tissues through a blowout fracture in the orbital floor.
- A horizontal fluid level indicating blood accumulation within the maxillary sinus is a sign of fracture.
- Sinus disease may cause opacification, but there will be no fluid level.

REFERENCE

1. Farber, S.J., Nguyen, D.C., Skolnick, G.B., Woo, A.S. and Patel, K.B. Current management of zygomaticomaxillary complex fractures: a multidisciplinary survey and literature review. *Craniomaxillofacial Trauma & Reconstruction* 2016;9(4):313–322.

SECTION 5
RADIOLOGICAL SIGNS OF ABUSE

13. SUSPECTED PHYSICAL ABUSE IN CHILDREN

More than 55,000 children were on child protection plans or registers in 2022 within the UK.[1] The Children Act 1989,[2] and subsequent additions to this, provides the legal framework for the safeguarding of children in England. This act allowed local authorities to 'make enquiries' if a child was suspected of being abused, but an amendment in 2004 dictated that all those who work with children are responsible for safeguarding them.[3] While radiographers will come across abusive injuries as part of a skeletal survey, on which they will not provide comment, they may come across suspicious appearances on images obtained for other reasons. It is therefore imperative that anybody looking at children's X-ray images can identify radiological signs that raise suspicions of abuse and follow local protocols for safeguarding.

Suspected physical abuse, previously known as non-accidental injury, is documented as far back as the mid 1800s, with clinicians linking suspicious post-mortem findings in children with physical punishment. The UK Crown Prosecution Service defines child abuse as being the infliction of harm or the failure to prevent harm to a child,[4] with harm being in the form of physical, emotional and/or psychological maltreatment, sexual abuse and/or neglect, which includes acts of omission. The Adoption and Children Act 2002 added the witnessing of domestic violence to this.[5] Given that fractures are the second most common presentation of abuse, it is generally the signs of physical abuse that radiographers are exposed to.[6]

For most attendances to the radiology department, it is normal to look at the clinical history and consider the abnormality that may be visualised on the images, such as an inversion injury leading to a possible lateral malleolus fracture. When abuse has taken place, this process needs to be reversed, as the presenting history may be limited or made up of falsifications intended to mislead clinicians. The images will speak for the victim; for example, a spiral fracture of the femur is caused by a twisting mechanism rather than a simple fall. When the abnormality is inconsistent with the given history, concerns must be raised with the referrer. If this is not possible, then a phrase must be added to the comment, for example 'injury not consistent with clinical information provided'.

While some of these injuries are extremely subtle and difficult to portray in a textbook, this chapter will attempt to shed some light on those appearances that raise concerns of abuse.

PATTERNS OF INJURY

Patterns of injury may differ depending on the child's age and the method of abuse. Under 2 years of age, metaphyseal and rib fractures are more common, along with head injuries, caused by the abuser gripping, shaking and throwing the child. Over this age, long bone fractures are more common. The radiological appearances that raise concerns fall into several categories.

Fractures of Long Bones in Children under the Age of 1 Year

A clear mechanism of injury is needed when a child under the age of 1 year presents with a fracture, as children of this age do not tend to fall over unless they are early walkers or are coasting around the furniture. Long bone fractures, either **transverse or spiral**, are the most common abusive fracture in children under 1 year, with the femur being the most common (**Figure 13.1**).[7] Spiral fractures have a greater association with abuse, as they are caused by a **twisting mechanism** and a child under the age of 1 year is unlikely to be able to generate enough force to cause such a fracture. The fracture can be subtle, and image magnification is often needed to identify it. **Defence fractures** in older children are also suspicious. These are fractures through the ulna shaft caused by raising the arm to protect the face and head from an incoming blow (**Figure 13.2a**).

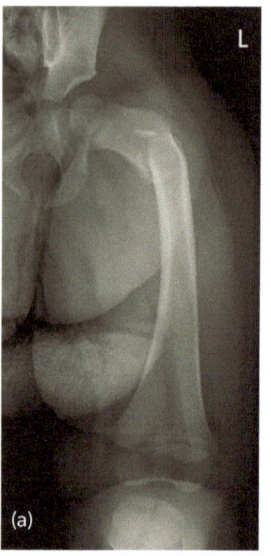 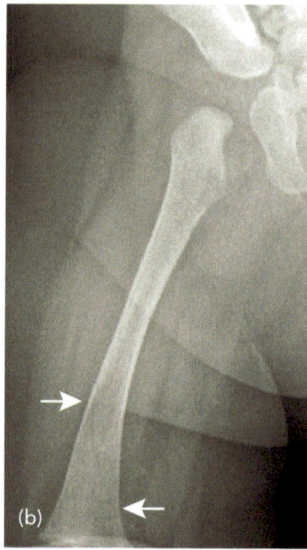

Figure 13.1 Anteroposterior femur images demonstrating (a) an angulated fracture through the proximal shaft and (b) a spiral fracture in a non-ambulant child.

Subperiosteal New Bone Formation (Periosteal Reaction)

Subperiosteal new bone formation can be an indication of fracture and is commonly seen in undisplaced traumatic spiral fractures of the tibia (see Figure 8.2b). However, the periosteum is loosely attached to the shaft of a child's long bone and if the limb is gripped hard then it can be lifted away, causing bleeding, which becomes visible as a **periosteal reaction** around 7 days later (**Figure 13.2**). If this is seen on an image, a mechanism of injury with a timeline is needed. It may be associated with a recent known injury, but if there is no reported trauma, for example, this could be an indication of abuse.

In children under the age of 6 months, there could be a **physiological (normal) subperiosteal new bone formation**, but this will be symmetrical, less than 2 mm thick and confined to the diaphysis.

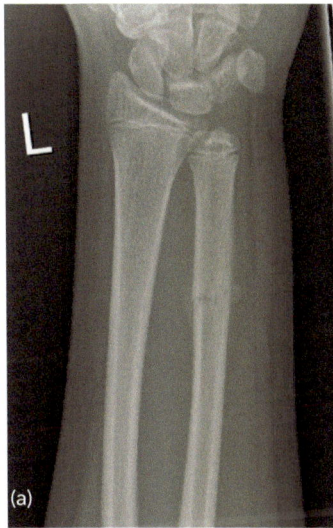
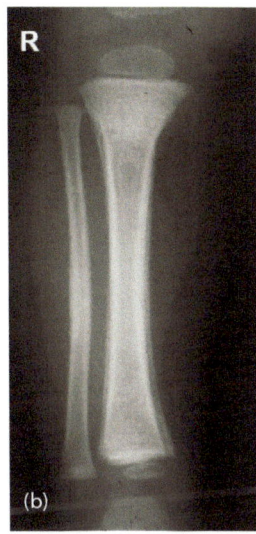

Figure 13.2 (a) Anteroposterior wrist image demonstrating a fracture through the distal ulna with a periosteal reaction. (b) Anteroposterior tibia and fibula with a periosteal reaction along the tibia and a healing fracture through the proximal tibia.

Healing and/or Multiple Fractures at the Time of Presentation

A fracture demonstrating signs of healing at initial presentation must raise suspicions of abuse (**Figure 13.3**). Correlation should be made between the image appearances and the presenting clinical history. It is possible to date most fractures by assessing the **stage of healing**, as outlined in Chapter 2, and this may enable the 'age' of the fracture to be determined. The stages of healing can be delayed if there is repetitive trauma or the child is malnourished. If there are **multiple fractures**, it is imperative that each separate fracture is dated to assist in the identification of ongoing abuse over a period of time. Figure 13.2b demonstrates a healing fracture in the proximal tibia with the fracture line no longer visible and hard callus formation, a process that takes up to 6 weeks in a child. In addition, this image also demonstrates a periosteal reaction through the lower tibia, a process that takes up to 3 weeks in a child, indicating that these are two separate injuries.

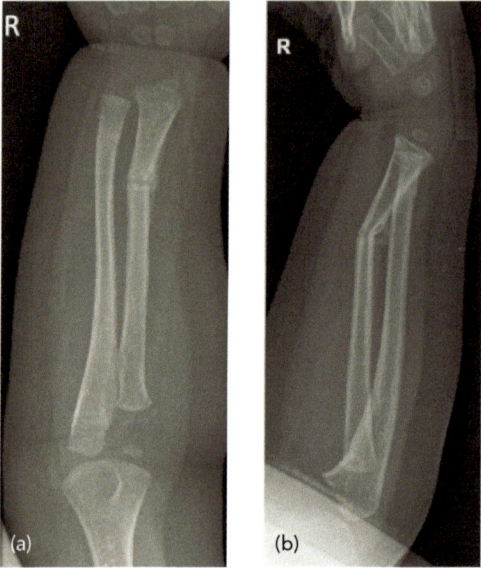

Figure 13.3 (a) Anteroposterior and (b) lateral forearm images demonstrating fractures to the distal radius and ulna showing signs of healing.

> **Comment:** fracture to the distal radius and ulna with posterior angulation at the radial fracture; signs of healing indicate this is not an acute injury.

Classical Metaphyseal Fracture

A metaphyseal fracture in a young child, without a clear mechanism of injury, is **pathognomic** of physical abuse. Unlike traumatic injuries, which generally occur as a buckle in the metadiaphyseal region, a classical metaphyseal fracture, also called a **corner fracture** or **bucket handle fracture** depending on its appearance, occurs immediately adjacent to the growth plate (**Figure 13.4**). Such fractures occur in children under the age of 2 years and are caused by a whiplash-type force being applied to the metaphysis in a flailing limb when a child is shaken. The periosteum is loosely attached in the diaphysis, but there is a strong attachment in the metaphysis. The flailing limb results in the periosteum avulsing a small fragment of bone.

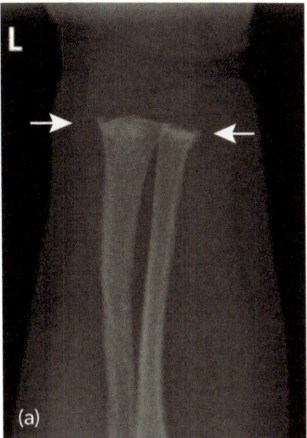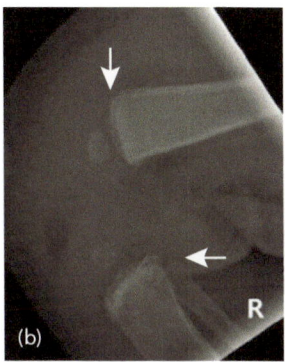

Figure 13.4 Different appearances of the classical metaphyseal fracture at the (a) distal radius and ulna and (b) distal femur and proximal tibia.

Skull Fracture under the Age of 2 Years

Skull X-ray following trauma is very rarely performed, as computed tomography (CT) is the imaging modality of choice; however, skull X-ray will be performed as part of a skeletal survey for suspected abuse. Normal development of the skull can cause some challenges in interpretation. There is the normal coronal, sagittal, lambdoid and squamosal sutures, but there are also the **mendosal** and **metopic** sutures visible. The mendosal suture lies in the occipital bone and the metopic suture lies in the frontal bone (**Figure 13.5**). Both close around the age of 6 to 7 years, but occasionally they persist into adult life and can be mistaken for a fracture. There are also numerous **synchondroses** in the base of the skull, which fuse around the age of 17 years. Sutures are non-linear lines measuring up to 10 mm wide at birth and are seen in very specific locations. A fracture has a linear appearance and can occur anywhere in the skull (**Figure 13.6**). The size of a skull fracture gives an idea of the cause. A traumatic fracture is likely to be less than 1 mm wide, as in Figure 13.6, but an abusive fracture tends to be greater than 2 mm wide because of the underlying raise in intra-cranial pressure (**Figure 13.7**).

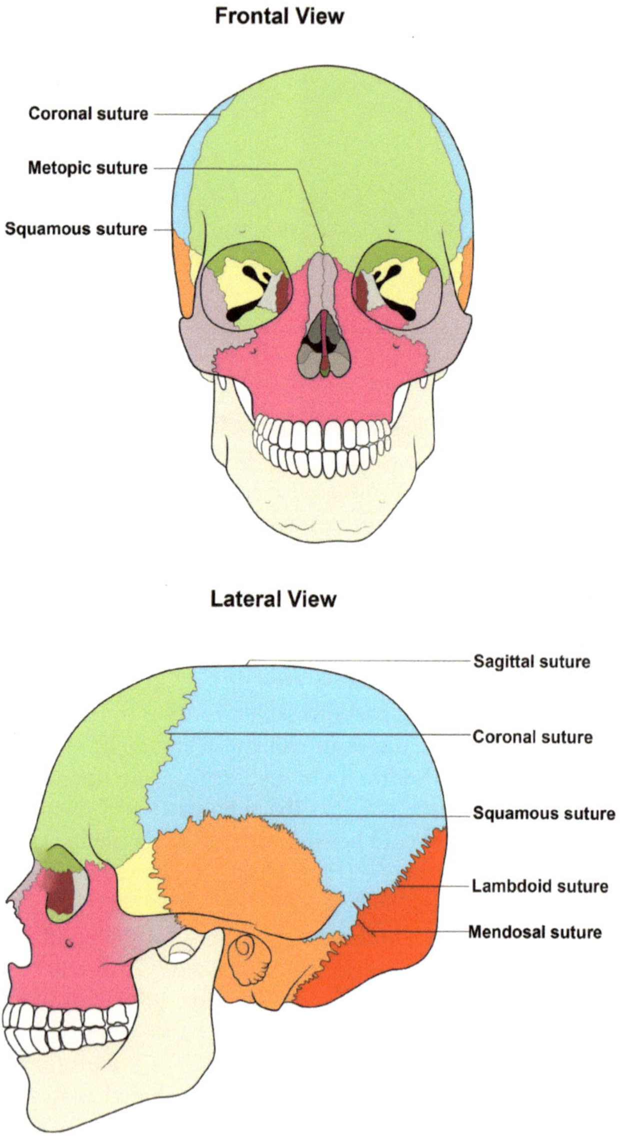

(a)

(b)

Figure 13.5 (a) Frontal and (b) lateral representations of the sutures.

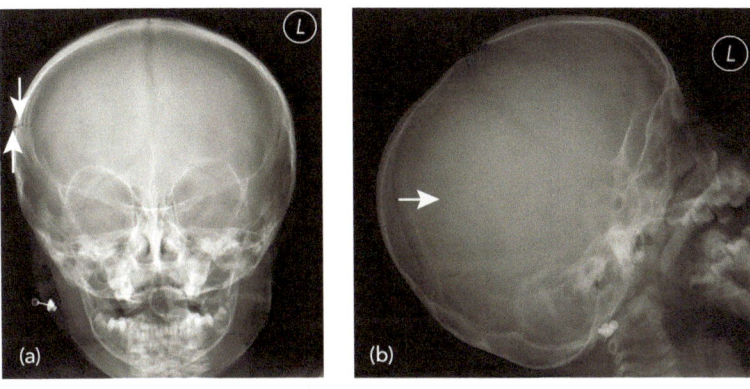

Figure 13.6 (a) Anteroposterior and (b) lateral skull images demonstrating a fracture in the right parietal bone.

Comment: fractured right parietal bone; clinical correlation required.

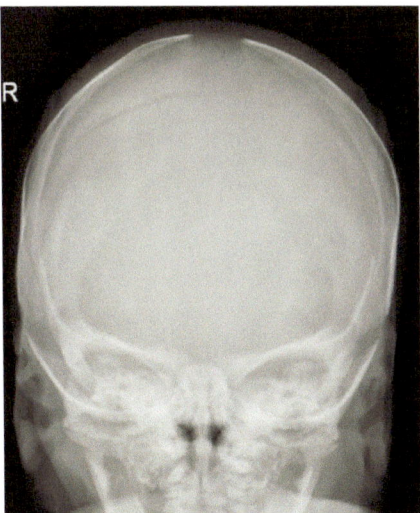

Figure 13.7 Townes skull image demonstrating significant widening of the sutures and a fracture in the right parietal bone.

Rib Fractures

There is much more to evaluate on a chest image than just the lungs. Rib fractures in children are almost always caused by abuse and may be discovered when a chest X-ray is performed for a simple cough or wheeziness. They occur in children under the age of 2 years, as they are caused by gripping the child around the chest while shaking them. This is not possible in older children, as they are able to punch and kick back. The compression forces applied by the adult fingers and thumbs cause fractures in the posterior ribs adjacent to the tubercle (**Figure 13.8**) and the anterior ribs adjacent to the costochondral junction. Fractures may not be visible on the initial image, and it is not uncommon to obtain an isotope bone scan if rib fractures are clinically suspected.

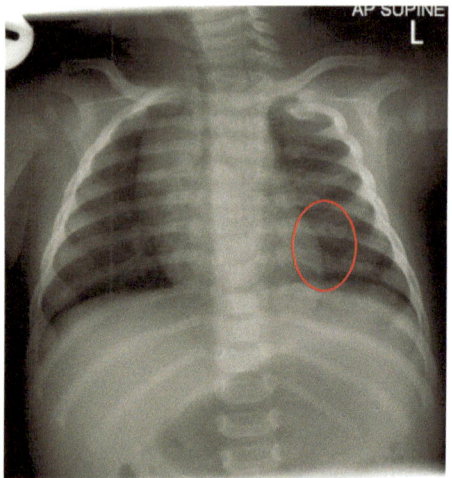

Figure 13.8 Anteroposterior supine chest image demonstrating left-sided rib fractures.

> **Comment:** fractures to the left seventh and eighth ribs; clinical correlation required.

UNUSUAL FRACTURES

Any fracture that occurs in an unusual position, such as in the spine, particularly at the cervicothoracic or thoracolumbar junction, should cause suspicion of abuse unless proven otherwise. Recognising radiological appearances and associated mechanisms of injury will help in determining if an abnormality identified on the images could possibly be caused by trauma.

CHAPTER SUMMARY

- When evaluating children's images, it is always important to keep in mind that some injuries are not accidental injuries.
- It is important to understand the mechanisms of injury for imaging appearances, and then to correlate these with the history given.
- Long bone fractures are the most common abusive fracture under the age of 1 year, with the femur being the most common of all long bones to be fractured.
- Although transverse fractures do occur in young infants as a result of abuse, spiral fractures caused by a twisting mechanism of injury are more common.
- A periosteal reaction or callus formation is evidence of delayed presentation and requires a clear mechanism of injury with a timeline that matches the radiological presentation.
- Metaphyseal fractures occur in children under the age of 2 years because of the whiplash-type force applied to this region.

REFERENCES

1. NSPCC. Child Protection Plan and Register Statistics: UK 2018–2022. 2023. Available at https://learning.nspcc.org.uk/media/os2k0rrh/child-protection-plan-register-statistics-uk-2018-2022.pdf.
2. Legislation.gov.uk. Children Act 1989. Available at https://www.legislation.gov.uk/ukpga/1989/41/contents.
3. Legislation.gov.uk. Children Act 2004. Available at https://www.legislation.gov.uk/ukpga/2004/31/contents.
4. Crown Prosecution Service Child Abuse (non-sexual). 2023. Available at https://www.cps.gov.uk/legal-guidance/child-abuse-non-sexual.
5. Legislation.gov.uk. Adoption and Children Act 2002. Available at https://www.legislation.gov.uk/ukpga/2002/38/contents.
6. Raynor, E., Konala, P. and Freemont, A. The detection of significant fractures in suspected infant abuse. *Journal of Forensic and Legal Medicine* 2018;**60**:9–14.
7. Leaman, L.A., Hennrikus, W.L. and Bresnahan, J.J. Identifying non-accidental fractures in children aged <2 years. *Journal of Children's Orthopaedics* 2016;**10**(4):335–341.

14. ABUSE OF OLDER PEOPLE

Older people are often vulnerable for several reasons, including a decline in mental and physical health. As a result, they may be unable to protect themselves and can fall victim to harm, generally from somebody who they trust.[1] Factors that make the identification of abuse of older people difficult include the following.

- **Neglect** and **acts of omission** are the most common forms of abuse, manifesting as poor personal and oral hygiene, a grubby appearance with overgrown toenails and untreated pressure sores.[2,3] This may also be the appearance of an older person who is attempting to maintain their independence but struggling to do so, rather than a neglectful act by a caregiver.
- Fracture risk is high, as older people may have lost bone density (**osteopenia**), making the bones more fragile, and they have reduced muscle mass (**sarcopenia**), leading to less protection around the bones. As a result, they can fracture a bone following relatively insignificant trauma, but this does not mean that they have been abused. While the most common sites for fracture following physical abuse are upper limbs, facial bones and posterior ribs, these can also be sites for traumatic injuries.
- Confused patients or those with **dementia** have an increased risk of fall and may also be unable to explain their injuries or they suggest a different mechanism of injury to that of the caregiver. While this could appear suspicious, it may be that they have simply had an unwitnessed fall. Care should be taken by the referring clinician to ensure that any discrepancy in the information being provided by the patient and caregiver is considered alongside the clinical and radiological findings[4] and that an unwitnessed fall is not a routine consideration for all unexplained injuries.[5]

Given these challenges, there is no surprise that the abuse of older people often goes unnoticed, with 95% of cases not being identified in an Emergency Department setting.[1] Radiographers are in a unique position. Radiation protection measures may result in the patient and carer becoming separated during imaging. Older people are often socially isolated and can be victims of abuse for significant periods of time before they meet somebody other than the abuser, so they may take this opportunity to **disclose abuse**.[6] **Figure 14.1** demonstrates fractures through the proximal phalanges following an alleged fall onto an outstretched hand; however, the patient disclosed abuse by the carer during imaging. In addition, during the imaging process, the radiographer may see physical signs of neglect or abuse if clothing needs to be removed. **Bruising** greater than 5 cm and found on the outside of the right arm, the face and the back is a common marker of abuse.[7] The correct local procedures for raising concern must be followed in these instances.

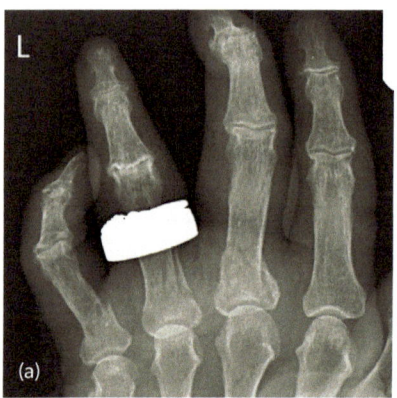 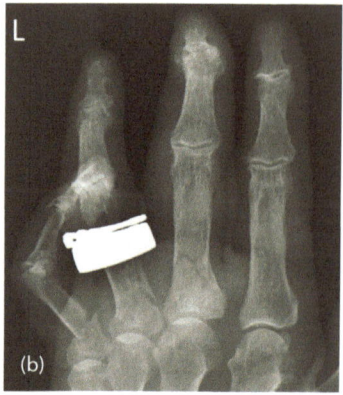

Figure 14.1 (a) Dorsi-palmar and (b) dorsi-palmar oblique images of the left hand demonstrating fractures through the proximal phalanges following an alleged fall onto an outstretched hand in a non-ambulant patient. The patient disclosed abuse by the carer during imaging.

Comment: fractures of the third to fifth proximal phalanges with posterior angulation at the fifth; the patient indicates that the mechanism is different from that provided on the referral.

RADIOLOGICAL APPEARANCES OF CONCERN

As with child abuse, inconsistent history and delayed presentation raise concerns of neglect or physical abuse. It is difficult to differentiate traumatic from non-traumatic injuries in older people. However, some radiological appearances raise suspicion of abuse and need to be recognised so that the clinician can explore the history and clinical presentation.

History Inconsistent with Image Appearances

Recognising radiological appearances and associated mechanisms of injury will help in determining if an abnormality identified on the images could have been caused by the given clinical history. Figure 14.1 demonstrates this; although the fractures could be traumatic and caused by a fall, given the disclosure by the patient they could also have been caused by forced hyperextension. It is essential that this disclosure is documented and raised with the referrer, following local procedures.

Healing Fracture at the Time of Presentation

Knowledge of **fracture healing processes** will assist in ageing any fracture (Chapter 2). If there are signs of an established healing process, then the history related to timing of the injury is essential (**Figure 14.2**). Fracture healing does take longer in older people due to the reduction in bone density, and this can also be affected by smoking, alcohol intake, poor diet and underlying illness. Periosteal reaction may be visible, but soft callus may not be visible until 6 weeks after trauma, with hard callus taking up to 6 months. It must be remembered that the fracture could have resulted from an unwitnessed accidental injury rather than an abusive injury; however, a delay in presenting with a non-independent older patient should raise concerns of neglect or an act of omission, as the patient may have been in pain or not using a limb and this was not addressed.

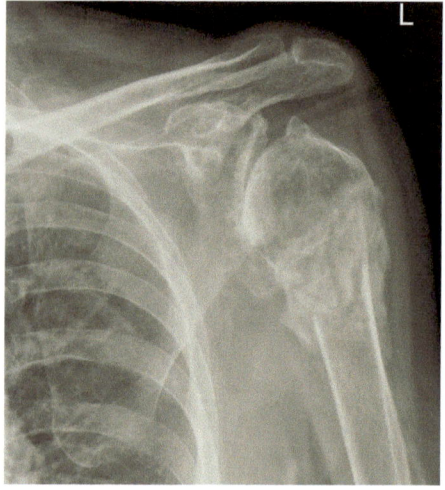

Figure 14.2 Anteroposterior shoulder image in a dementia patient presenting with a fall the previous day and demonstrating a healing fracture through the proximal humerus with disorganised callus formation due to lack of immobilisation at the time of injury.

Facial Bone Fractures

Accidental falls in older people generally result in upper or lower limb injuries and midface fractures involving the nasal bones, orbits and zygoma.[8] They are likely to also have associated bruising. The lack of extremity injury or other bruising when a patient presents with isolated facial bone injuries should raise concern, especially if the injury involves the **left zygoma, orbit or maxilla**.[8] A punch by a right-handed person will inflict left-sided injuries (**Figure 14.3**).

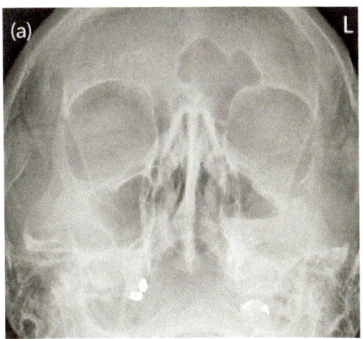 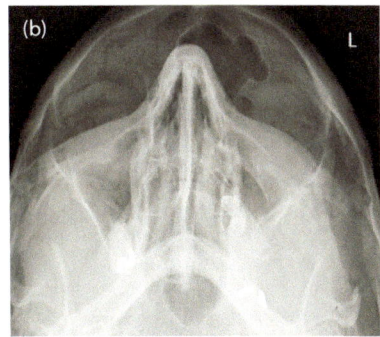

Figure 14.3 (a) Occipitomental and (b) occipitomental 30° facial bone images demonstrating injuries to the left zygomaticomaxillary complex and a left maxillary sinus fluid level.

> **Comment:** fractures of the left orbital floor and zygoma; widened left frontozygomatic suture; fluid level left maxillary sinus; correlate clinically.

CHAPTER SUMMARY

- A patient may disclose abuse during the imaging examination. Follow the appropriate safeguarding procedures.
- Fractures that do not correlate with the clinical history may be abusive and a false clinical history may have been provided to cover up abuse.
- Fractures that are healing at the time of presentation may be accidental; however, failure to take an older patient for appropriate care may be an act of omission or neglect.
- Some fractures may appear accidental but have a higher significance in older people and an abusive injury should be considered.

REFERENCES

1. NHS Digital. Safeguarding Adults Collection, Annual Report, England 2016–17. 2017. Available at https://digital.nhs.uk/data-and-information/publications/statistical/safeguarding-adults/2016-17.

2. Murphy, K., Waa, S., Jaffer, H., Sauter, A. and Chan, A. A literature review of findings in physical elder abuse. *Canadian Association of Radiologists* 2013;**64**:10–14.

3. Wigglesworth, A., Austin, R., Corona, M. and Mosqueda, L. Bruising as a forensic marker of physical elder abuse. *Journal of the American Geriatrics Society* 2009;**57**(7):1191–1196.

4. Faircloth, E. Elder abuse: our responsibilities in society and healthcare. *Imaging and Oncology* 2016:10–15.

5. Wong, N.Z., Rosen, T., Sanchez, A.M., Bloemen, E.M., Mennitt, K.W., Hentel, K. et al. Imaging findings in elder abuse: a role for radiologists in detection. *Canadian Association of Radiologists* 2017;**68**(1):16–20.

6. Rosen, T., Hargarted, S., Flomenbaum, N.E. and Platts-Mills, T.F. Identifying elder abuse in the emergency department: toward a multidisciplinary team-based approach. *Annals of Emergency Medicine* 2016;**68**(93):378–382.

7. Ziminski, C.E. Injury patterns and causal mechanisms of bruising in physical elder abuse. *Journal of Forensic Nursing* 2013;**9**(2):84–91.

8. Rosen, T., Lofaso, V.M. and Bloemen, E.M. Identifying injury patterns associated with physical elder abuse: analysis of legally adjudicated cases. *Annals of Emergency Medicine* 2020;**76**:266–276.

SECTION 6
PATHOLOGICAL FINDINGS WITHIN THE MUSCULOSKELETAL SYSTEM

15. COMMENTING ON ARTHRITIS

When evaluating images of the skeleton, one element of the review is the cartilaginous areas, which include the joints. There are many pathological conditions affecting the joints and, while it is not the purpose of the person providing a comment on the images to diagnose these conditions, it is important to recognise when a joint does not demonstrate normal characteristics. Any joint disease is referred to as an **arthropathy**, and any arthropathy can result in **arthritis**. Technically, the term arthritis is an overarching term used to describe inflammation within the joint. This chapter will focus on the most common forms of arthritis:

- degenerative arthritis, also called **osteoarthritis (OA)**, which is mainly age-related and therefore occurs in most people;
- inflammatory arthritis, which is a result of an underlying systemic illness in which the body's own defence system attacks the tissues of the joints. The most commonly occurring inflammatory arthropathies are **rheumatoid arthritis (RA)**, **gout** and **ankylosing spondylitis**.

Different arthritides can present with their own classical radiological appearances, but there are some similarities too:

- changes in bone density, such as increased **periarticular lucency** or **subchondral sclerosis**;
- loss of joint space;
- loss of alignment with atraumatic subluxations or dislocations;
- loss of bone at the articular surfaces or increased bone proliferation;
- increased thickness of soft tissues around the joints.

It is important to recognise that, when a joint is damaged by disease, it quite often leads to OA, as the normal function of that joint is affected. This means that a single joint may demonstrate multiple pathologies. While it is not essential to comment on all appearances of arthritis, consideration must be given to the presenting history and the patient's age. If the presenting history relates to pain associated with a joint, and if that joint has appearances suggestive of arthritis, then it is perhaps prudent to comment on this, as this is likely to be the cause of the pain. If a younger patient presents following trauma and changes associated with arthritis are noted on the images, then this too must be commented on, as it is unusual to see such arthritic changes in younger age groups.

JOINT ANATOMY

Before looking at the different pathologies affecting the joints, a brief look at the anatomy of a synovial joint should assist in understanding disease development and the subsequent radiological appearances. A synovial joint is a fluid-filled joint contained within a joint capsule and is the most common joint in the human body (**Figure 15.1**). The capsule has a fibrous outer layer, which is continuous with the periosteum, and a synovial inner layer (**synovium**). The synovium secretes **synovial fluid**, which acts as a lubricant for the joint. The articular surfaces of the associated bones making up the joint are covered in a thin layer of **hyaline cartilage**, which acts as a shock absorber. Many synovial joints have **bursae**, which are small synovial fluid-filled sacs located in the parts of the skeleton where there will be high levels of friction during movement. Diseases that affect the joints generally have an impact on the articular cartilage and synovial fluid, causing reduction in joint space.

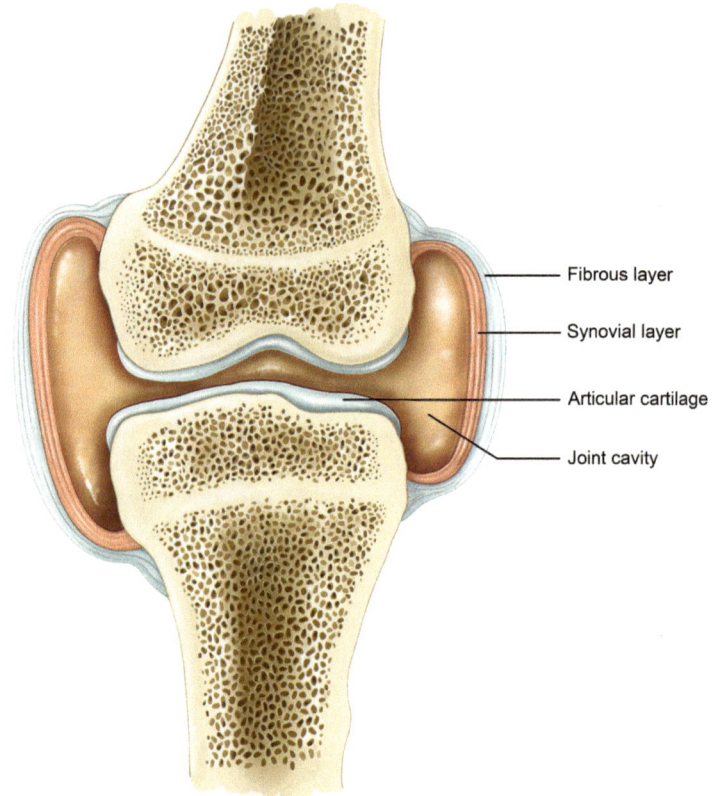

Figure 15.1 Synovial joint anatomy.

DEGENERATIVE ARTHRITIS

Osteoarthritis

OA is a degenerative disease affecting much of the adult population. There are many contributory factors, but the most common is age-related wear and tear, referred to as **primary OA**. The disease is distributed asymmetrically, with the knee being the most affected joint, followed by the hips and the hands. Other factors include previous joint injury or the presence of another joint arthropathy, such as infection, and this is referred to as **secondary OA**. This can occur in any joint and at any age.

There is variable correlation between the radiological appearances of OA and the presenting symptoms, so somebody with very few symptoms can have significant changes within the joint. Typical radiological appearances of OA include (**Figure 15.2**):

- joint space **narrowing** caused by deterioration in the articular cartilage;
- **osteophyte** formation caused by the subchondral bone remodelling, resulting in marginal bony spurs;
- **subchondral sclerosis** caused by thickening of the subchondral bone;
- **subchondral cyst formation** caused by the intrusion of synovial fluid through cracks in the articular cartilage and subchondral bone;
- deformity within the adjacent bony contours caused by **subchondral bone loss**;
- loss of joint alignment caused by **ligamentous instability**.

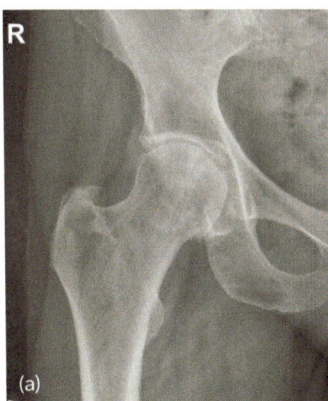 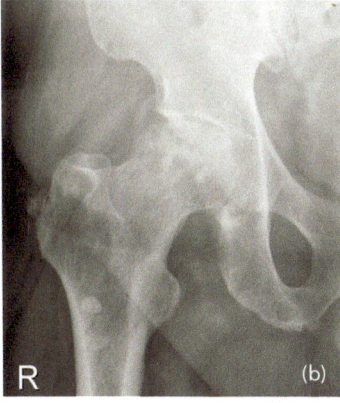

Figure 15.2 Anteroposterior hip images demonstrating (a) mild signs of OA and (b) severe signs of OA.

Femoroacetabular impingement can also lead to early OA. This presents as a painful hip with limited range of movement. It is a form of developmental anomaly in which there is overgrowth of bone at the acetabulum (pincer lesion) (Figure 15.3) or the femoral head is unusually shaped (cam defect) (Figure 15.4).

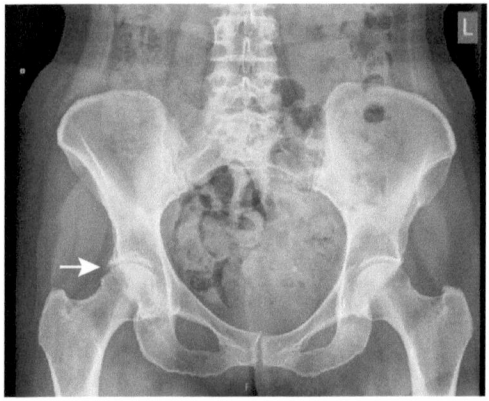

Figure 15.3 Anteroposterior pelvis image demonstrating a right-sided pincer lesion and mild OA in the right hip.

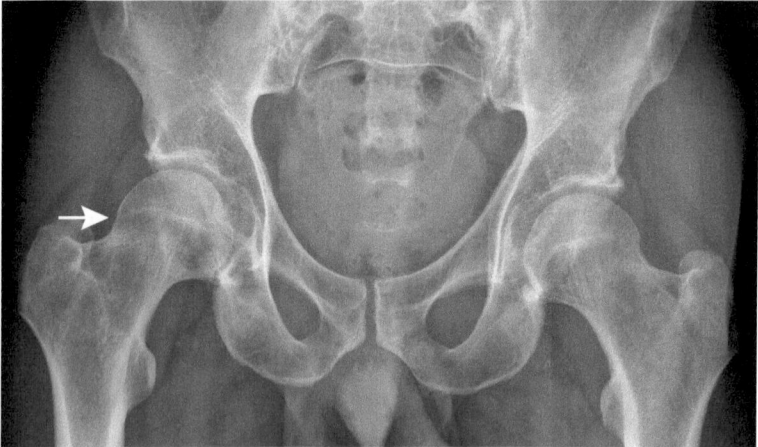

Figure 15.4 Anteroposterior hips demonstrating mild bilateral degeneration and a right-sided cam defect. Compare the femoral necks; the junction between the head and neck on the right looks like a slope; this is the cam defect.

A form of OA that affects the hands of post-menopausal females is **erosive OA**. The distal interphalangeal joints are affected most, but it can also be found in the proximal interphalangeal joints (**Figure 15.5**). In addition to the normal characteristics of OA, erosive OA has central erosions within the phalangeal head, producing an appearance that is often likened to a **gull wing**.

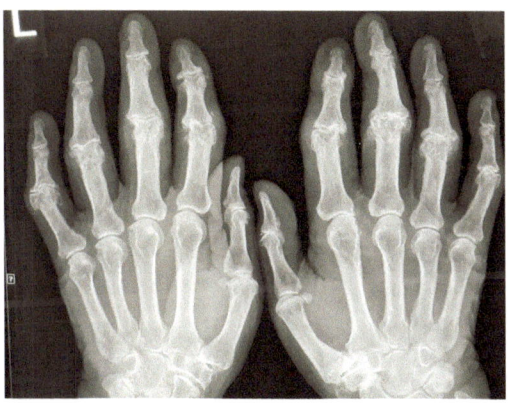

Figure 15.5 Dorsi-palmar image of both hands demonstrating erosive OA.

> **Comment: joint space loss at numerous interphalangeal joints with central erosions and some degenerative subluxations.**

Degenerative Disease of the Spine

Degenerative disease in the spine, often referred to as **spondylosis**, has the same appearances as in other joints. While the intervertebral disc spaces are fibrocartilaginous joints, the facet joints are synovial joints, and increased **facet sclerosis** is often the first sign of spinal degeneration. Degenerative disease of the spine causes reduced intervertebral disc spaces, **end plate sclerosis** and osteophytes, which develop horizontally (**Figure 15.6**). As the disease progresses, there may be loss of alignment of the vertebral bodies. If the appearance shows the osteophytes becoming joined to each other (i.e. running vertically) but the intervertebral disc space maintains its normal height, this is **diffuse idiopathic skeletal hyperostosis (DISH)**, in which the anterior longitudinal ligament ossifies (**Figure 15.7**), giving the appearance of flowing oste-ophytes. The differentiating factor between spondylosis and DISH is the intervertebral disc space, which retains its normal height in DISH but is reduced in height in spondylosis. A further similar appearance is **syndesmophytes**, which will be discussed later in this chapter.

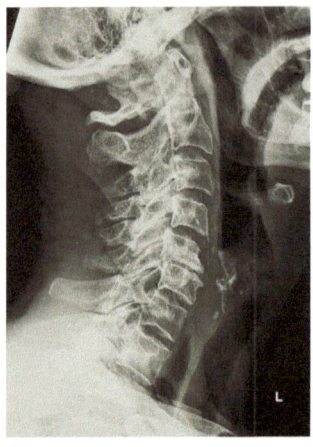

Figure 15.6 Lateral cervical spine image demonstrating moderate degeneration.

Comment: reduction at the C5/6 intervertebral disc space with osteophytes. Facet sclerosis. Retrolisthesis of C5. Prevertebral soft tissues are normal.

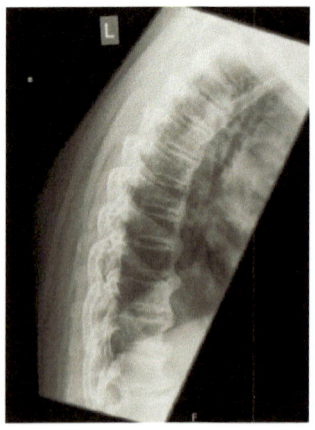

Figure 15.7 Lateral thoracic spine image demonstrating diffuse idiopathic skeletal hyperostosis.

INFLAMMATORY ARTHRITIS

Rheumatoid Arthritis

RA is a chronic autoimmune inflammatory disorder in which there is erosion of the bones making up a joint. There is abnormal proliferation of the synovial membrane leading to a thickened synovium (**pannus**). The pannus invades the bone, which is not protected by articular cartilage (the bare points) and causes **erosions (Figure 15.8)**. It also destroys the cartilage, leading to joint space loss. Osteoclastic activity in the juxta-articular regions outweighs osteoblastic activity because of hyperaemia (increased blood flow) leading to juxta-articular osteopenia. The patient will present with the typical arthritic symptoms of pain, stiffness and swelling, but in addition they may also have warmth and tenderness around their joints. As this is a systemic illness, they

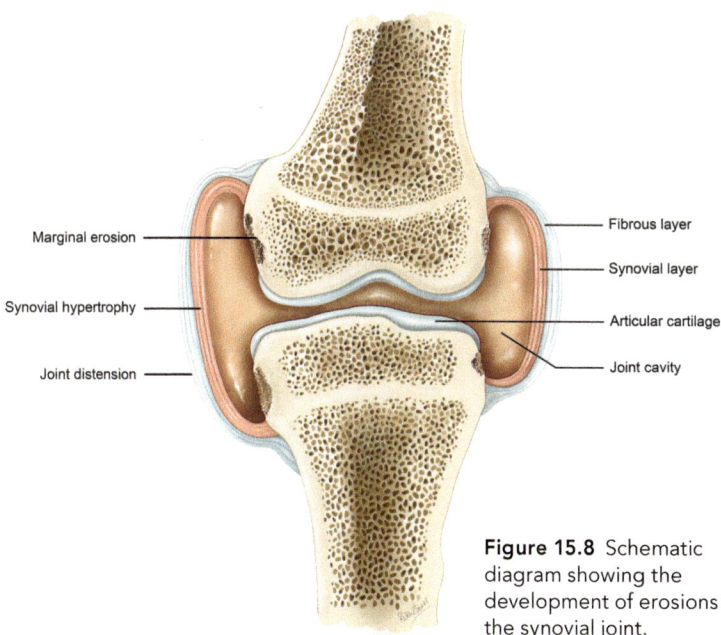

Marginal erosion

Synovial hypertrophy

Joint distension

Fibrous layer

Synovial layer

Articular cartilage

Joint cavity

Figure 15.8 Schematic diagram showing the development of erosions in the synovial joint.

may also demonstrate fatigue and fever, with reduction in appetite resulting in weight loss. The joint pain tends to be worse in the morning and improves as the day goes on. The patient may also have other signs of rheumatoid arthritis, such as a skin rash, uveitis (redness in the eyes) or neuropathy.

The classical radiological appearances include:

- juxta-articular osteopenia;
- loss of joint space;
- periarticular erosions;
- soft tissue swelling from nodular thickening of the tendon sheath leading to flexion deformities;
- joint destruction/subluxation;
- ankylosis of the small joints of the hands and feet;
- no evidence of sclerosis or osteophytosis unless secondary OA is present.

Unlike OA, radiological distribution of RA is symmetrical. The small joints of the hands and feet are affected initially and, if left untreated, larger joints such as the hips, elbows and shoulders may also be affected. In the hands, early disease commonly affects the proximal interphalangeal joints, the metacarpophalangeal joints and the ulna styloid process (**Figure 15.9**). In the feet, early disease commonly affects the metatarsophalangeal joints (**Figure 15.10**).

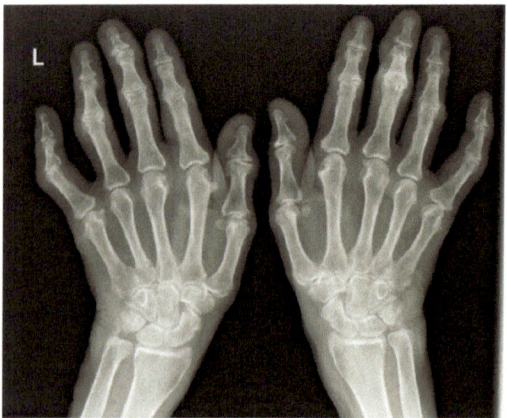

Figure 15.9 Dorsipalmar hands image demonstrating erosions at numerous proximal interphalangeal and metacarpophalangeal joints bilaterally and the left ulna styloid process.

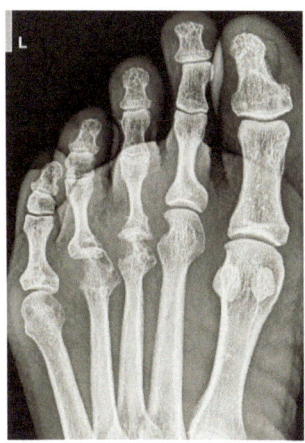

Figure 15.10 Dorsi-plantar toes image demonstrating erosions at the metatarsophalangeal joints.

Juvenile idiopathic arthritis is the most common inflammatory condition in the paediatric skeleton. This presents as inflammation within the joints, and the radiological appearances are like those associated with RA in adults. However, the impact on the growing skeleton can be immense, with premature fusion of the physis, resulting in limb length discrepancies.

Ankylosing Spondylitis

Ankylosing spondylitis classically presents in young patients as severe back pain, often initially over the sacroiliac joints, which improves with exercise and deteriorates overnight. The initial radiological appearances are in the sacroiliac joints, with initial bilateral widening of the joints before they narrow and develop iliac sclerosis (referred to as **sacroiliitis**) and erosions (**Figure 15.11**). As the disease progresses, the sacroiliac joints fuse and will be difficult to visualise. On lateral spine imaging, there may be the appearance of fine vertical osteophytes; however, these are not related to the horizontal osteophytes previously discussed within degeneration of the spine. These are **syndesmophytes**, which are formed when the anterior longitudinal ligament or annulus fibrosus calcifies. If this appearance is evident at multiple levels, then it is classical for ankylosing spondylitis (**Figure 15.12**).

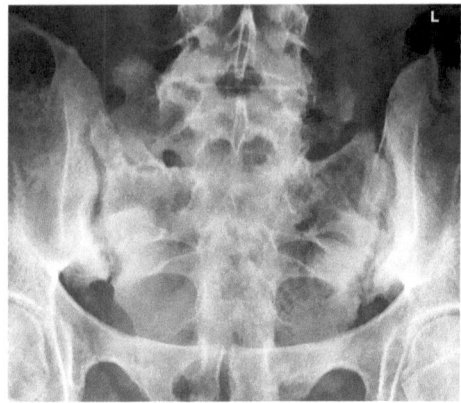

Figure 15.11 Posteroanterior sacroiliac joints demonstrating increased sclerosis and widening indicating sacroiliitis.

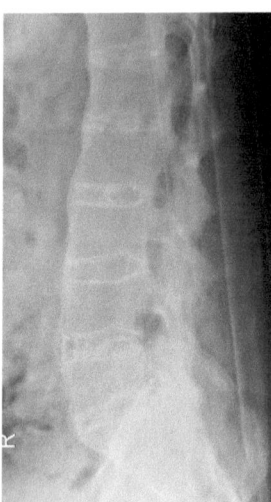

Figure 15.12 Lateral spine image demonstrating ankylosing spondylitis.

Gout

Gout most commonly affects the big toe, although it can occur in other joints, and presents as sudden onset of intense pain. It is caused by an accumulation of uric acid crystals within the joint space, which leads to inflammation and eventually to bone destruction. A classical appearance of gout is as a **punched-out lesion** with overhanging edges at the periphery of the articular surface (**Figure 15.13a**). This is often accompanied by an increase in adjacent soft tissue density because of a **tophus**, formed when the uric acid crystals deposit within the soft tissues (**Figure 15.13b**). Gout can be differentiated from RA by the overhanging edge of the lesion and the lack of periarticular osteopenia.

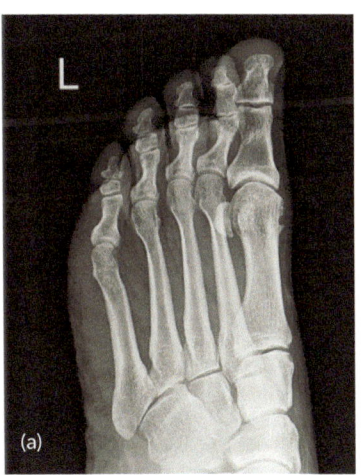 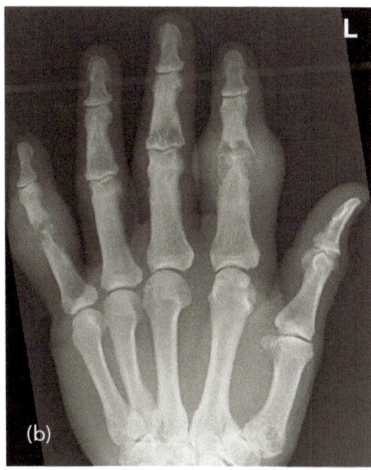

Figure 15.13 (a) Dorsi-plantar oblique foot image demonstrating a punched-out lesion with overhanging edges on the first metatarsal head and (b) dorsi-palmar oblique hand image demonstrating gouty arthritis and soft tissue tophi at the second and fifth proximal interphalangeal joints. There is also OA at the first carpometacarpal joint.

CHAPTER SUMMARY

- Primary OA is age related.
- Secondary OA is related to an underlying condition that has affected the normal articulation of the joint.
- Radiological appearances of OA are joint space narrowing, osteophyte formation, subchondral sclerosis and subchondral cyst formation.
- Erosive OA has the normal signs of OA and has central erosions.
- Femoral acetabular impingement is a form of developmental anomaly in which there is a pincer lesion or a cam defect.
- Osteophytes in the spine are seen in the horizontal plane.
- Syndesmophytes in the spine are seen in the vertical plane and are related to ankylosing spondylitis.
- Inflammatory arthritis is a result of an underlying systemic illness in which the body's own defence system attacks the tissues of the joints.
- The radiological appearances of RA are juxta-articular osteopenia, loss of joint space, periarticular erosions and, in the later stages, joint destruction/subluxation and ankylosis.
- Gout leads to juxta-articular erosions with a punched-out appearance and overhanging edges. There may also be increased soft tissue density over the joint, called a tophus.

16. COMMENTING ON INFECTION

Patients with a musculoskeletal infection will present with a range of symptoms, including pain, swelling, redness, erythema and warmth at the infected site. It is extremely important to identify radiological signs of infection and make sure that this is mentioned in the comment, as infection in bones or the joint spaces can have devastating consequences. A magnetic resonance imaging scan is more sensitive to musculoskeletal infective changes than X-rays, but there are some signs to be vigilant of when evaluating X-ray images. In most cases, loss in bone density, seen as focal **osteopenia**, is seen in the early stages. When osteopenia is adjacent to the articular surface, recognising whether the focus of infection is in the bone or the joint is important. An infection in the bone will demonstrate focal osteopenia, which does not cross the joint, but an infection within the joint will demonstrate symmetry in the osteopenia on both sides of the joint. However, it must be recognised that 30% of actual bone density must be lost before it becomes apparent on an X-ray image. The most common bone infection is **osteomyelitis**, and the most common joint infection is **septic arthritis**. Osteomyelitis close to a joint can lead to septic arthritis, so the two pathologies may be seen alongside each other. These will be discussed in detail within this chapter.

Acute and chronic changes will have different appearances, and these can be compounded by other pathologies; for example, an infection can occur in an arthritic joint and an arthritic joint can be caused by previous infection. Identifying all of the pathologies is essential for the clinician in determining the most appropriate onward management.

OSTEOMYELITIS

Osteomyelitis is by far the most common bone infection, caused by the *Staphylococcus* bacteria commonly found on the surface of the skin. If there is a break in the skin, then the bacteria can reach the underlying bone. This may be through a traumatic or a surgical wound. It can also be because of **vascular compromise**, as seen in patients with peripheral vascular disease or diabetes mellitus. Raised pressure within the compromised veins causes damage to the small vessels, leading to fragile skin that easily lacerates. This, with the added risk of impaired skin healing, can result in an ulcer forming. Once infection has entered through a skin wound, it is able to attach itself to the underlying bone. Image appearances follow a typical pattern but, in the early stages of the infection, they can be very subtle.

- Soft tissue swelling is likely to be present along with changes within the fat planes or lucencies within the soft tissues associated with **pockets of gas** produced by the bacterial infection (**Figure 16.1**).
- Osteopenia will develop at the site of the infection, and this may appear as a focal lucency around implanted metalwork if the infection is associated with a surgical implant (**Figure 16.2**).
- There will be a periosteal reaction (Figure 16.2).
- Left untreated, there will be focal bone loss with rapid deterioration seen over subsequent images.

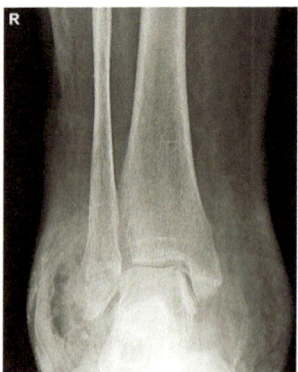

Figure 16.1 Anteroposterior ankle image demonstrating soft tissue swelling and extensive gas within the soft tissues laterally. There is also focal osteopenia and loss of clarity at the cortex of the lateral malleolus indicating osteomyelitis.

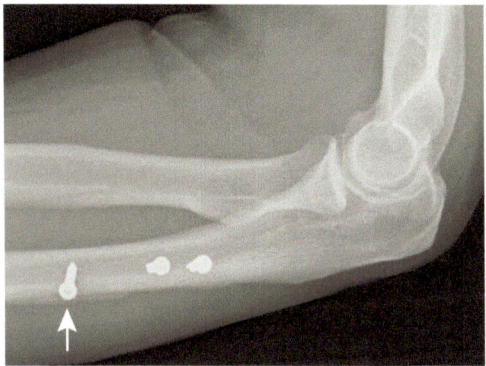

Figure 16.2 Lateral image of an elbow demonstrating lucency and periosteal reaction associated with the distal screw.

If antibiotic therapy is successful, there will be peripheral sclerosis at the site of the bone loss and no further damage will be caused. However, if the infection does not respond to antibiotic therapy, further bone loss will be seen and a sequestrum and involucrum may develop.

- A sequestrum is a small fragment of bone that has become separated and displaced from the site of infection as the bone starts to break down (**Figure 16.3**).
- An involucrum is a layer of new bone that develops around the sequestrum.

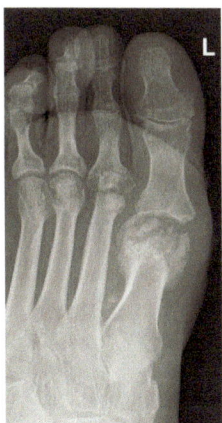

Figure 16.3 Dorsi-plantar toes image demonstrating a sequestrum at the head of the first metatarsal.

Chronic osteomyelitis can lead to the need for surgical amputation if conservative treatment including antibiotics is not successful in slowing down the progression of disease.

Occasionally, the infection may be caused by bacteria travelling through the bloodstream from a remote source of infection, such as a urinary tract infection, and depositing within the bone (**haematogenous spread**). This is more common in children under the age of 5 years due to the slow rate of blood flow in the metaphyseal region, and in older people with underlying conditions such as peripheral vascular disease. Haematogenous spread in adults, while less common, tends to result in **vertebral osteomyelitis**, sometimes referred to as **discitis**, although this condition can also occur following an intervention, such as surgery or lumbar puncture.

Vertebral Osteomyelitis

Vertebral osteomyelitis is caused most commonly by *Staphylococcus aureus*. It generally starts in the end plate of the vertebral body and progresses into the intervertebral disc space. Early diagnosis is essential in preventing significant and devastating damage to the spine. The initial presentation is of excruciating back pain with red flag signs of fever or reduced appetite. X-ray images taken in the early stages are likely to be normal. However, once the infection has become established, radiological signs of narrowing of the intervertebral disc space and irregularity with bone loss at the associated end plates should raise suspicions of vertebral osteomyelitis (**Figure 16.4**).

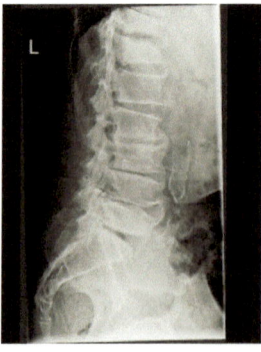

Figure 16.4 Lateral lumbar spine image demonstrating the impact of vertebral osteomyelitis at T11/12 along with degenerative changes elsewhere and aortic calcification.

Brodie's Abscess

Brodie's abscess is a subacute form of osteomyelitis that presents as an interosseous abscess predominantly in the metaphyseal region of long bones in children. While they have similar aetiology to osteomyelitis, as described above, the radiological appearance can present a confusing picture. The initial appearance is of an oval lucent lesion orientated along the long axis of a long bone (**Figure 16.5**). There is generally a dense sclerotic rim and there may be a lucency extending through the sclerotic rim in the direction of the growth plate. This latter appearance is what differentiates a Brodie's abscess from any other lesion. Periostitis and soft tissue swelling may also be present.

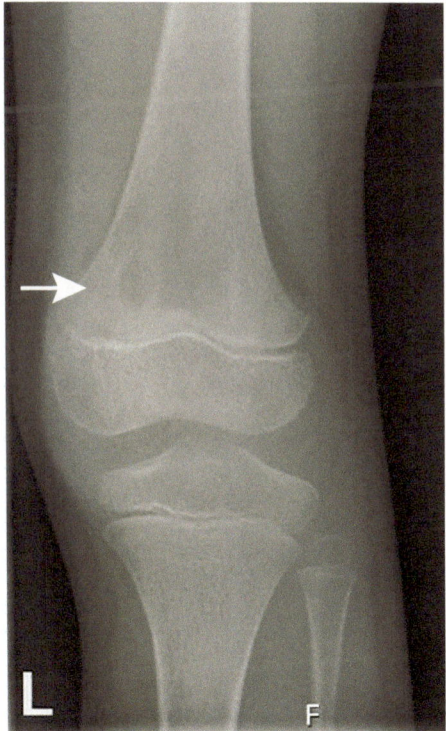

Figure 16.5 Anteroposterior knee image demonstrating a Brodie's abscess in the distal femur.

SEPTIC ARTHRITIS

Like any other arthritis, septic arthritis involves inflammation within the joint space. The inflammation is caused by an infection that has entered the joint capsule through a direct route or more commonly through the blood supply to the joint. Haematogenous infections are more common in children and in older patients; the presence of a joint replacement, for example in an older patient, increases the risk of infection being introduced into the joint. The most common bacteria responsible for septic arthritis is *Staphylococcus aureus*. Depending on the time to presentation, the initial imaging can be normal, as it does take some time for the radiological appearances to become apparent. Infection in a joint may demonstrate joint space widening before the joint space reduces, caused by damage to the articular cartilage. This is followed by juxta-articular osteopenia and bone loss on either side of the joint (**Figure 16.6**).

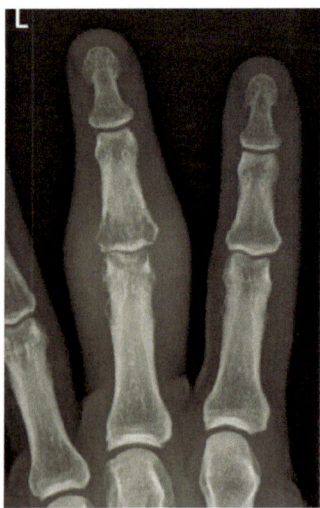

Figure 16.6 Dorsi-palmar finger image demonstrating soft tissue swelling and juxta-articular osteopenia at the proximal interphalangeal joint of the middle finger.

CHAPTER SUMMARY

- Osteomyelitis is most common in the diabetic foot, and care must be taken to produce diagnostic images and to identify early signs to prevent future significant consequences.
- Early radiological signs of osteomyelitis can be subtle and changes within the soft tissues, such as soft tissue swelling or gas collections, are suspicious.
- Other signs of osteomyelitis include elevation of the periosteum, focal osteopenia and bone destruction.
- Osteomyelitis and septic arthritis can have similar appearances, but the differentiating factor is the appearance in relation to the joint space. As septic arthritis starts within the joint, osteopenia and bone destruction will be apparent within the bones either side of the joint.

17. COMMENTING ON BONE LESIONS

Bone lesions are formed when normal bone is replaced with abnormal bone or tissue. They can be lucent (lytic), sclerotic or mixed; singular or multiple; and benign or aggressive. Bone lesions are referred to as 'aggressive' rather than 'malignant', with the latter being a term associated with cancer, as aggressive lesions can encompass non-cancerous pathologies such as osteomyelitis, discussed in Chapter 16. Any bone lesion puts the bone at risk of a fracture, referred to as a **pathological fracture**, and this may be the first presentation of a bone lesion. They can also be associated with several syndromes.

There are many bone lesions, each with their own unique identifiers but also with many similarities. It is not the role of the radiographer to interpret the radiological appearances and offer a diagnosis, but it is the role of the radiographer to recognise those that do not need immediate input and those that require urgent escalation. The **zone of transition** is one of the more important radiological differentiators. This is the interface between the normal bone and the abnormal bone and is described as being narrow or wide.

- A narrow zone of transition indicates a non-aggressive, or benign, lesion. There may be a sclerotic border around the lesion, but occasionally the sclerotic border will not be present. If you can draw a line around the lesion, then you can be confident in suggesting that this is a benign lesion.
- A wide zone of transition indicates an aggressive lesion. The border between normal and abnormal bone is not easy to see and you cannot draw a line around the lesion.

In addition to the zone of transition, other factors to consider when evaluating images in which there is a bone lesion are the appearances of the cortex and the periosteum. A lesion that results in destruction of the cortex or an associated periosteal reaction (**periostitis**) is usually an aggressive lesion and will need an urgent report. Follow local procedures for making sure that the image is acted on urgently. This chapter will look at the more common bone lesions and expand on these findings.

BENIGN BONE LESIONS

Benign bone lesions do not necessarily need expediting for urgent report, but if there is any concern about the features of a lesion it is always sensible to seek advice from a reporting practitioner before allowing the patient to leave the department.

Non-ossifying Fibroma

A non-ossifying fibroma is a lucent lesion within the cortex of a bone and is a common incidental finding in the metaphyseal region of the distal tibia and the distal femur in children. As the child grows, the lesion migrates away from the metaphysis, so it may be seen in the metadiaphysis or, less commonly, the diaphysis. The lesion has a narrow zone of transition with a thin sclerotic border, but it may be multiloculated, the cortex may be thinned but not destroyed, and it does not have a periosteal reaction (**Figure 17.1**). Non-ossifying fibromas can grow to a reasonable size, but they are self-limiting lesions that resolve without any clinical input. During the resolution stage, the lesion may appear sclerotic.

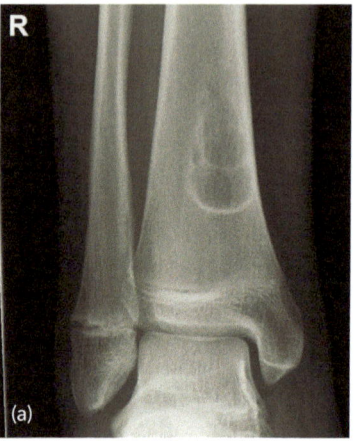 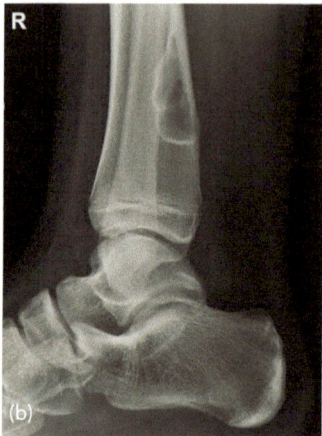

Figure 17.1 (a) Anteroposterior and (b) lateral ankle images demonstrating a non-ossifying fibroma.

> **Comment:** well-defined lucent lesion, distal tibia; no fracture; normal alignment.

Simple Bone Cyst

Also referred to as a **solitary bone cyst** or a unicameral bone cyst, this is a fluid-filled cavity that develops within the bone and is seen as a lucent lesion in children and adolescents, most commonly in the meta-diaphyseal region of the proximal humerus or proximal femur. It may be in contact with the growth plate and, in this instance, this is an **active** simple bone cyst, which will continue to grow. A simple bone cyst that is not in contact with the growth plate is said to be **latent**. The size of the cyst is likely to remain constant and, as the long bone grows, the distance between the cyst and the growth plate will increase. The patient may present following an insignificant trauma that has resulted in significant pain, and a pathological fracture may be evident on imaging. Radiologically, a simple bone cyst presents as an area of increased lucency with a narrow zone of transition and thin sclerotic margin. There may be expansion of the cyst with some thinning of the adjacent cortex, although the cortex is not breached unless a pathological fracture occurs. If a fracture does occur through this weakened portion of bone, a bone fragment may be visible within the cyst, and this is referred to as a **fallen fragment sign** (**Figure 17.2a**).

Aneurysmal Bone Cyst

An aneurysmal bone cyst consists of a loculated blood-filled lesion that has a narrow zone of transition and a sclerotic border (**Figure 17.2b**). Unlike a simple bone cyst, the patient may present with symptoms of pain and swelling caused by the increasing size of the lesion. Aneurysmal bone cysts are typically found in the metaphysis of long bones but can appear anywhere in the skeleton. Due to the expanding nature of this type of lesion, it can result in cortical breach.

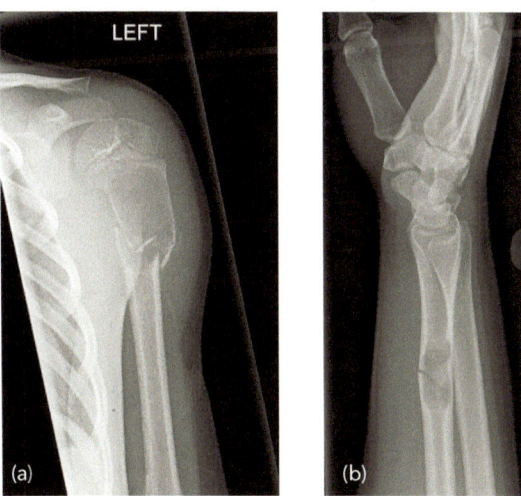

Figure 17.2 Pathological fractures demonstrated in (a) an anteroposterior proximal humerus with a simple bone cyst and (b) a lateral distal radius with an aneurysmal bone cyst.

Enchondroma

This is perhaps the most common benign bone lesion. It is often found in the fingers, but can also present in the diaphysis of any bone (**Figure 17.3**). Like a solitary bone cyst, this is usually an incidental finding and may only become apparent following an injury that results in a pathological fracture. Radiologically, it is an area of lucency with a narrow zone of transition and a thin sclerotic margin. It can appear expansile without breaching the cortex, but the cortex does become thinned and can easily fracture. The lesion can sometimes have a ground glass appearance and demonstrate some internal calcifications.

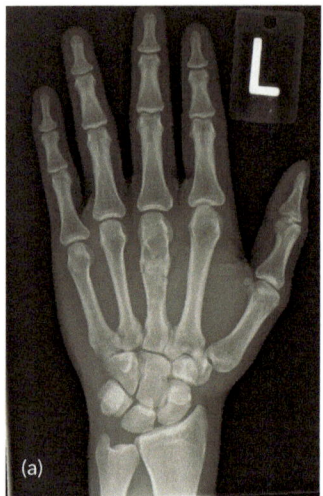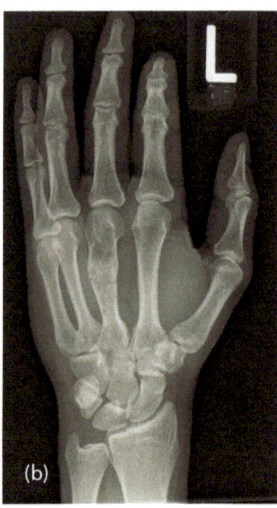

Figure 17.3 (a) Dorsi-palmar and (b) dorsi-palmar oblique hand images demonstrating a fracture through an enchondroma.

> Comment: **fracture in the third metacarpal through a well-defined lucent lesion.**

Giant Cell Tumour

This is a benign lucent lesion; it is locally aggressive in the speed at which it grows, so it does have a narrow zone of transition, but there will be absence of the sclerotic border. It has similar appearances to another benign lucent bone lesion, a **chondroblastoma**, and the difference between them is the patency of the growth plate. For a diagnosis of giant cell tumour the growth plate is fused, and for a diagnosis of chondroblastoma the growth plate is patent. The giant cell tumour is located eccentrically in the metaphysis of a long bone and abutting the articular surface (**Figure 17.4**). As the lesion grows, it may thin and then breach the cortex. While this is a benign lesion, there may be a periosteal reaction visible.

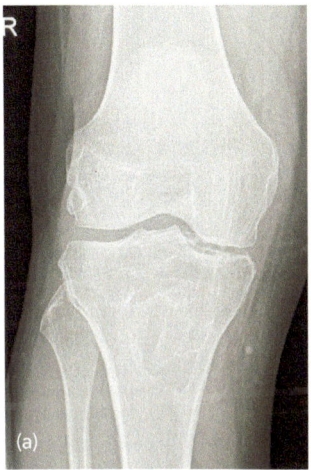 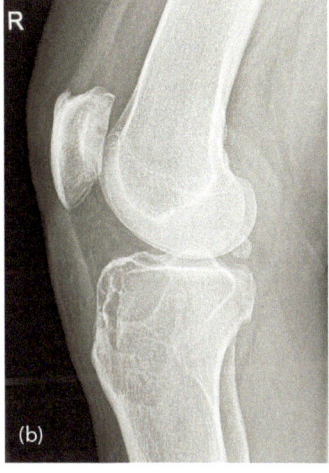

Figure 17.4 (a) Anteroposterior and (b) lateral knee images demonstrating a giant cell tumour.

> **Comment: large defined lucent lesion in the proximal tibia. No fracture. Normal alignment.**

Osteochondroma

An osteochondroma is a common benign bone lesion (**Figure 17.5**). Such lesions are often an incidental finding unless they are large and cause impingement upon adjacent nerves or vessels, in which case the patient will present with pain. They commence in the metaphyseal region of the bone in the second decade of life and migrate away from the growth plate as the child grows. There are two radiological presentations of an osteochondroma:

1. a **broad-based (sessile)** osteochondroma has a wide base, and the cortex and medulla of the normal bone follow the line of the osteochondroma;
2. a **pedunculated** osteochondroma has a stalk.

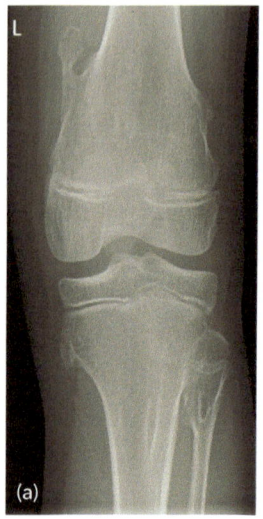

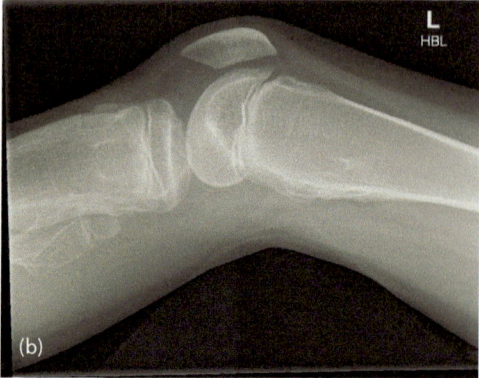

Figure 17.5 (a) Anteroposterior and (b) lateral knee images demonstrating multiple osteochondromas; a pedunculated osteochondroma is seen on the medial femur and broad-based osteochondromas are seen on the lateral femur, fibula neck and medial tibia.

> **Comment:** no fracture, normal alignment. Multiple benign lesions (osteochondromas).

Both variants have a **cartilaginous cap**, which is usually less than 3 cm in a child and can be negligible in an adult when seen on a magnetic resonance scan. While the osteochondroma itself is a benign lesion, the cartilaginous cap can undergo malignant transformation. The signs that this may be occurring include an increase in the size of the cartilaginous cap, further growth of the osteochondroma after skeletal maturity or localised aggressive features. Some patients may have **multiple osteochondromas**. An **exostosis**, or a bone spur, has a similar appearance but does not have a cartilage cap.

Osteoid Osteoma

An osteoid osteoma is a benign sclerotic lesion occurring predominantly in the femur and tibia in children. The presenting complaint will be severe pain at night, which is relieved by aspirin or non-steroidal anti-inflammatory medication, and it will most likely lead to an atraumatic limp. Radiologically, this lesion presents as a defined dense area of thickened cortex that can be expansile (**Figure 17.6**). It contains a central area of lucency called a **nidus**, which differentiates this lesion from any other. If the central nidus is greater than 2 cm then a benign osteoblastoma should be considered, although this is most often seen in the spine. Osteoid osteoma in the spine often leads to scoliosis and this diagnosis should always be considered when a patient presents with scoliosis.

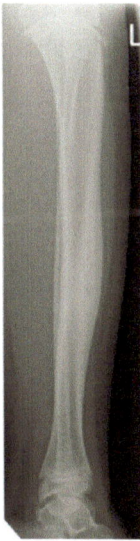

Figure 17.6 Lateral tibia and fibula image demonstrating an osteoid osteoma.

AGGRESSIVE LESIONS

The most common aggressive bone lesions seen outside specialist orthopaedic centres are **myeloma** and **metastatic disease**. These must be considered in any patient over the age of 40 years who presents with a lucent or a sclerotic bone lesion. The most common primary bone tumours are **osteosarcoma** and **Ewing's sarcoma**, both seen in younger patients under the age of 25 years. A wide zone of transition is the earliest appearance of an aggressive lesion, and it may also have endosteal scalloping and periostitis. While it is sensible to seek advice on any lesion seen on images, a lesion that demonstrates aggressive features must be expedited for urgent report. It may be that the lesion is known about, but progression of disease must be assessed by a reporting practitioner.

Myeloma

Myeloma is a cancer of the **plasma cells**. It can be benign, showing no clinical or radiological signs, but if a blood test indicates the presence of myeloma cells, then regular follow-up is needed, as the disease can progress to multiple myeloma, which is aggressive and can spread from the bone into adjacent soft tissues or into other organs through blood and lymphatic systems. Radiologically, the lesions are seen as small round lucencies that have a narrow zone of transition but no sclerotic margin and scalloping within the endosteum if the lesion is close to it (**Figure 17.7**).

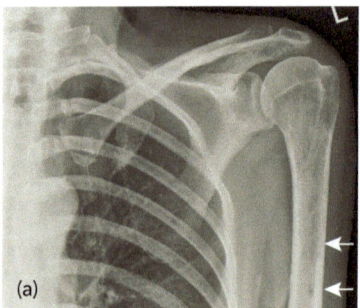 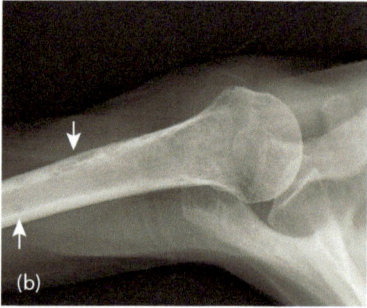

Figure 17.7 (a) Anteroposterior and (b) axial shoulder images demonstrating multiple small lesions from myeloma.

> **Comment:** no fracture; normal alignment; multiple lucencies in the proximal humerus.

Metastases

Bone metastases can be lucent, sclerotic or a mixture of the two. Lucent metastases look like myeloma in the early stages and radiological differentiation can be difficult. Metastatic lesions have a wide zone of transition and will breach the cortex as they grow. They are also at risk of a pathological fracture (**Figure 17.8**). They may also develop a periosteal reaction, something which is not commonly seen in myeloma. Metastases are rarely seen in the distal extremities.

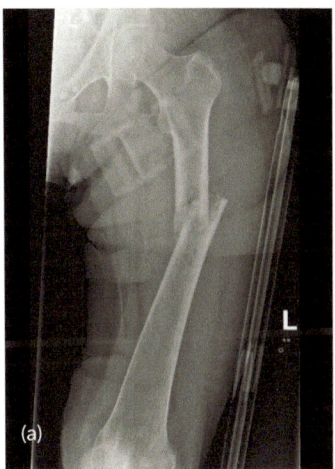 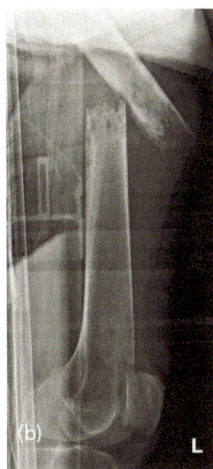

Figure 17.8 (a) Anteroposterior and (b) lateral images of a proximal femur demonstrating a pathological fracture through an aggressive lesion. Note the wide zone of transition and the irregularity of the fracture margins.

> **Comment: fracture of the midshaft of the femur with medial angulation and posterior displacement, through an aggressive-looking lesion.**

Breast and **prostate cancer** are the most common types of cancer in the UK and these both metastasise to bone, with breast metastases being mixed lucent and sclerotic and prostate metastases commonly being sclerotic (**Figure 17.9**). There may be several lesions, and their aggressive nature will result in cortical destruction and may lead to pathological fracture.

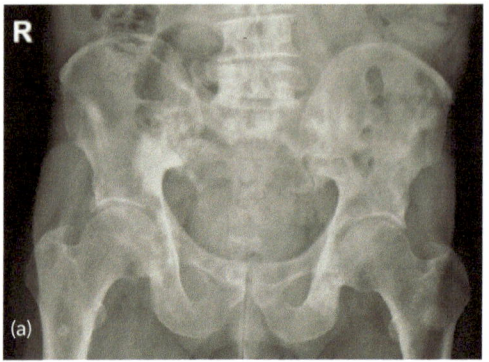

Comment: multiple sclerotic lesions throughout the pelvis; mild degeneration of the hips.

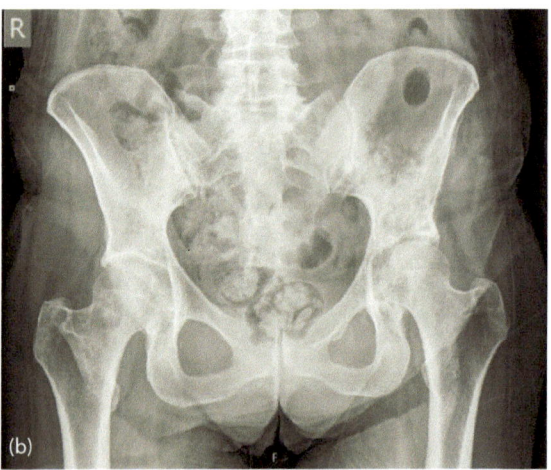

Comment: lucent lesion in the right femoral neck, mixed lesion with aggressive features in the left acetabulum and ilium.

Figure 17.9 Anteroposterior pelvis images demonstrating (a) sclerotic metastatic deposits throughout the pelvis and proximal femora and (b) a mixed lesion in the left acetabulum and ilium, and a lucent lesion in the right femoral neck.

Osteosarcoma

Osteosarcoma is the second most common tumour affecting bone in the older population and the first most common bone tumour in children. It is found in the intramedullary region of long bones. Radiologically, the lesion will have the typical aggressive appearances of a wide zone of transition, bone destruction and periosteal reaction (**Figure 17.10a**). As the lesion progresses, it will extend into the adjacent soft tissues.

Ewing's Sarcoma

Ewing's sarcoma is the second most common bone tumour in children, seen most often in the metadiaphysis of long bones, but also in the pelvis and shoulder. Radiologically, this has typical aggressive appearances, with bone destruction, a permeative ('moth-eaten') appearance, periostitis and a wide zone of transition. Soft tissue extension is often also present (**Figure 17.10b**).

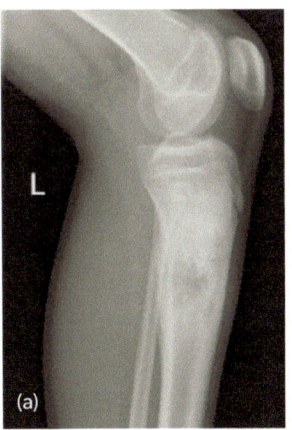
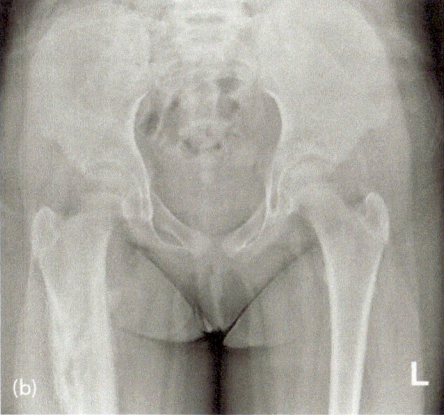

Figure 17.10 (a) Lateral knee image demonstrating an osteosarcoma. (b) Anteroposterior pelvis image demonstrating a Ewing's sarcoma of the right femur.

CHAPTER SUMMARY

- The zone of transition is important in differentiating between a benign and an aggressive lesion.
- A benign bone lesion will demonstrate a narrow zone of transition without a break in the cortex unless that is a pathological fracture. Benign bone lesions do not necessarily need expediting for urgent report, but, if there is any concern about the features of a lesion, it is always sensible to seek advice from a reporting practitioner before allowing the patient to leave the department.
- An aggressive bone lesion will demonstrate a wide zone of transition and may also have endosteal scalloping, periosteal reaction and cortical bone destruction. These lesions must be expedited for urgent report.
- Myeloma and metastases have similar appearances; however, metastatic lesions have a wide zone of transition, can breach the cortex and can develop a periosteal reaction.
- Aggressive lesions can develop a soft tissue component.

SECTION 7
PRACTICE CASES

18. PRACTICE CASES

It is difficult in a text such as this to include subtle findings, as image reproduction removes some of the resolution that is available on viewing monitors, imaging tools are not available for manipulation and the images are only small. Images with obvious deformities have been used as the focus of this chapter, which is an opportunity to practise using the knowledge and skills gained throughout the previous chapters and to apply this to the development of a comment on a range of images.

Look at the images presented and review the short clinical history before using the small section for notes to help gather your thoughts. Alternatively, templates are available in Chapter 1, which can be copied and used to support your evaluation and comment development.

Once you have looked at the images and reached your own conclusion, a detailed, structured approach to the evaluation is presented. This will enable you to explore your own thought processes further, measured against those of an experienced reporting practitioner. Finally, an appropriate comment is suggested using the templates presented in Chapter 1.

PRACTICE CASE 1

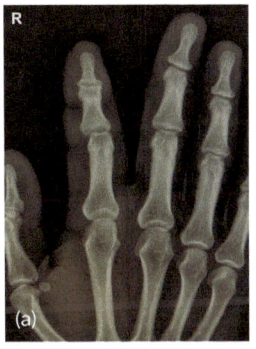 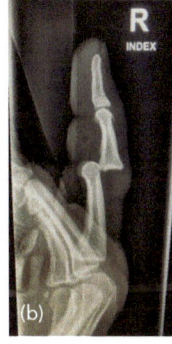

Figure 18.1 (a) Dorsi-palmar and (b) lateral index finger images for evaluation following a fall, with deformity to the index finger.

Notes:

_____

_____

_____

_____

_____

Table 18.1 Experienced reporting practitioner's detailed evaluation.

Thought process following the ABCs systematic method of evaluation	
Adequacy	The images are adequate.
Bones	The cortices are intact and there are no areas of abnormal density.
Cartilaginous areas	The joint space at the proximal interphalangeal joint of the index finger is widened on the dorsi-palmar image. On the lateral image, the middle phalanx has moved posteriorly, and the articular surfaces are not congruous. This is a posterior dislocation – remember to describe the direction of the distal aspect.
	The distal interphalangeal joint is slightly reduced on the lateral image, but alignment is satisfactory. There is an osteophyte on the dorsal aspect of the middle phalanx at this joint. When looking on the dorsi-palmar image, it is difficult to see the distal interphalangeal joint because of flexion caused by the deformity at the proximal interphalangeal joint, but there are signs of degeneration visible.
Soft tissues	The soft tissues are grossly swollen.

Developing the comment		
A	Abnormality type	Dislocation
B	Bone details	No fracture
C	Cartilage involvement	Second proximal interphalangeal joint
D	Displacement	Posterior
E	Extra features	Soft tissue swelling and degeneration at the distal interphalangeal joint

Writing the comment

Second proximal interphalangeal joint dislocation with posterior displacement and soft tissue swelling. Note, it is not necessary to also comment on the degenerative features, as they are only mild and likely age related.

PRACTICE CASE 2

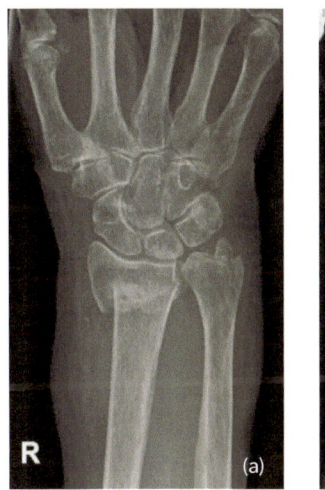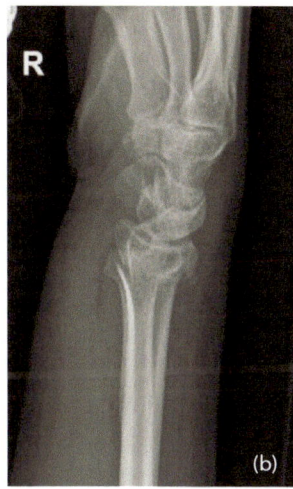

Figure 18.2 (a) Dorsi-palmar and (b) lateral wrist images for evaluation following a fall onto the outstretched hand, with deformity and bruising to the wrist.

Notes:

_____

_____

_____

_____

_____

Table 18.2 Experienced reporting practitioner's detailed evaluation.

Thought process following the ABCs systematic method of evaluation	
Adequacy	The images are adequate to answer the clinical question.
Bones	There is a transverse, extra-articular fracture through the distal radius, but close inspection shows that it is comminuted, as there is a separate fracture fragment on the dorsal aspect. It is also angled dorsally and there is a small degree of impaction. In addition, the ulnar styloid process is fractured.
Cartilaginous areas	Alignment of the carpus is normal. There is disruption of the joint space at the distal radio-ulna joint, but this is caused by the dorsally angulated radial component of the joint.
Soft tissues	Soft tissues are swollen, and the pronator quadratus fat stripe is displaced.

Developing the comment		
A	Abnormality type	Fracture
B	Bone details	Distal radius and ulna styloid process
C	Cartilage involvement	While the radial fracture involves the distal radio-ulna joint, the main radiocarpal joint is not affected. The ulna styloid process fracture is intra-articular as is always the case
D	Displacement	Dorsally angulated distal radius
E	Extra features	Comminuted distal radius

Writing the comment
Fracture through the distal radius, which is dorsally angulated and comminuted, and a fracture of the ulna styloid process.

PRACTICE CASE 3

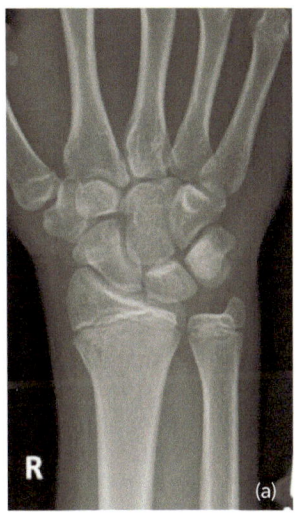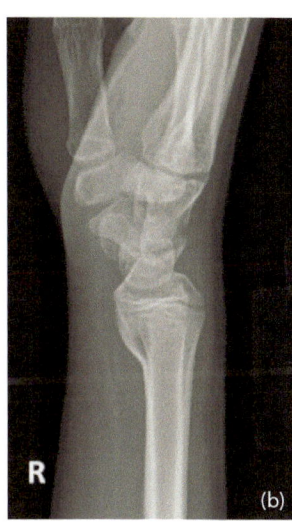

Figure 18.3 (a) Dorsi-palmar and (b) lateral wrist images for evaluation following a fall onto the outstretched hand, with painful wrist.

Notes:

_____

_____

_____

_____

_____

Table 18.3 Experienced reporting practitioner's detailed evaluation.

Thought process following the ABCs systematic method of evaluation	
Adequacy	The images are adequate to answer the clinical question.
Bones	There is disruption in the lateral metaphysis of the distal radius on the dorsi-palmar image and in the anterior cortex on the lateral image. The opposing cortex on both images is intact, suggesting that this is not a transverse fracture and it likely extends to the distal radial growth plate.
Cartilaginous areas	Radiocarpal alignment is normal and the carpal arcs are intact.
Soft tissues	The pronator quadratus fat stripe is elevated.

Developing the comment		
A	Abnormality type	Fracture
B	Bone details	Distal radius metaphysis
C	Cartilage involvement	No involvement of the joints but the fracture extends to the growth plate
D	Displacement	No displacement
E	Extra features	None

Writing the comment
Fracture through the anterolateral metaphysis of the distal radius extending to the growth plate (Salter–Harris type II).

PRACTICE CASE 4

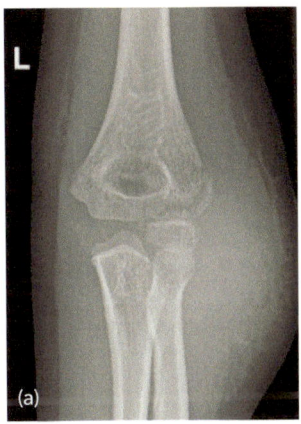 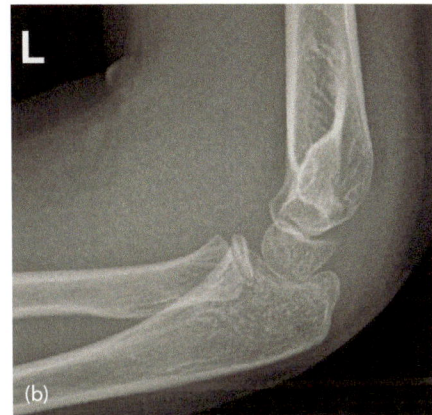

Figure 18.4 (a) Anteroposterior and (b) lateral elbow images obtained following a fall onto the outstretched hand.

Notes:

_____

_____

_____

_____

_____

Table 18.4 Experienced reporting practitioner's detailed evaluation.

Thought process following the ABCs systematic method of evaluation	
Adequacy	The images are adequately positioned and the exposure is appropriate for bone and soft tissue.
Bones	There are two bony fragments next to the lateral condyle of the humerus. Using knowledge of ossification around the elbow, the capitellum, radial head and internal epicondyle can be seen, but the trochlea and olecranon cannot be seen. Therefore, it is extremely unlikely that the second fragment represents the ossification centre of the external epicondyle. This is a unicondylar fracture of the external condyle.
Cartilaginous areas	The head of the radius is articulating normally with the capitellum, as indicated by the radiocapitellar line. The anterior humeral line passes through the middle third of the capitellum. The fracture line extends to the growth plate.
Soft tissues	There is gross soft tissue swelling to the lateral elbow and an elbow joint effusion.

Developing the comment		
A	Abnormality type	Fracture
B	Bone details	Distal humerus – lateral (external) condyle
C	Cartilage involvement	Extends to the growth plate
D	Displacement	Minimal distraction
E	Extra features	Gross soft tissue swelling

Writing the comment	
	Unicondylar fracture of the lateral condyle reaching the growth plate, with gross soft tissue swelling.

PRACTICE CASE 5

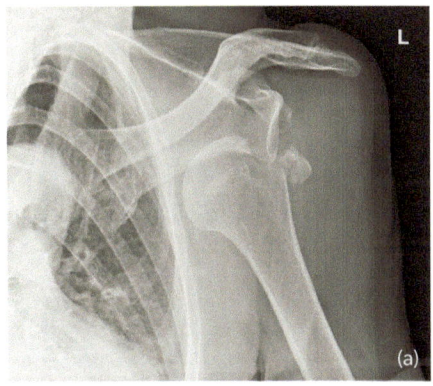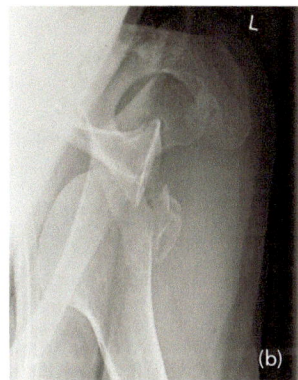

Figure 18.5 (a) Anteroposterior and (b) axial shoulder images obtained following a fall onto the outstretched hand.

Notes:

_____

_____

_____

_____

_____

Table 18.5 Experienced reporting practitioner's detailed evaluation.

Thought process following the ABCs systematic method of evaluation	
Adequacy	The images are diagnostically acceptable.
Bones	There is irregularity at the greater tuberosity with fragmentation. The remaining bones appear intact.
Cartilaginous areas	The head of the humerus has displaced from the glenoid cavity and is sitting underneath the coracoid process indicating an anterior dislocation of the glenohumeral joint (GHJ).
	Acromioclavicular and sternoclavicular alignment appear to be within normal limits.
Soft tissues	Looking within the lung fields, lung markings can be seen to the periphery of the chest cavity.
	No lesions are visible.

Developing the comment		
A	Abnormality type	Fracture dislocation
B	Bone details	Greater tuberosity comminuted fracture
C	Cartilage involvement	GHJ joint dislocation
D	Displacement	Distraction at the fracture. Anterior displacement at the GHJ
E	Extra features	None

Writing the comment
Anterior dislocation of the GHJ with a comminuted fracture of the greater tuberosity.

PRACTICE CASE 6

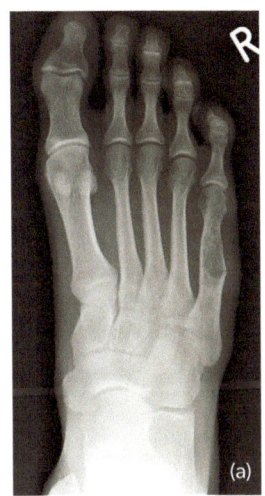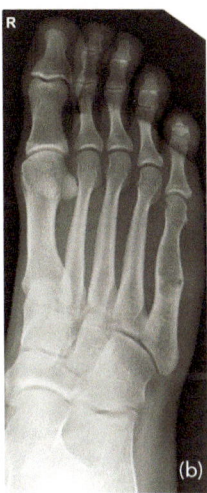

Figure 18.6 (a) Dorsi-plantar and (b) oblique foot images obtained following an inversion injury while playing football.

Notes:

_____

_____

_____

_____

_____

Table 18.6 Experienced reporting practitioner's detailed evaluation.

Thought process following the ABCs systematic method of evaluation	
Adequacy	The images are adequate and a diagnosis can be made.
Bones	There is a lucency in the midshaft of the fifth metatarsal that has a narrow zone of transition but looks slightly expansile. The cortex is thinned with a little bit of scalloping but there is no periosteal reaction, and the lesion does not have any aggressive features. The most common benign lucency in a metatarsal is an enchondroma. There is a lucent line extending through this lesion but not breaching the medial cortex. This represents a pathological fracture.
Cartilaginous areas	The joint spaces are preserved, and the fracture does not extend to the articular margin.
Soft tissues	There is a small amount of soft tissue swelling adjacent to the fracture.

Developing the comment		
A	Abnormality type	Fracture
B	Bone details	Midshaft of the fifth metatarsal
C	Cartilage involvement	None visible
D	Displacement	None
E	Extra features	Benign lucent lesion

Writing the comment
Fracture to the midshaft of the fifth metatarsal through a benign lucent lesion.

PRACTICE CASE 7

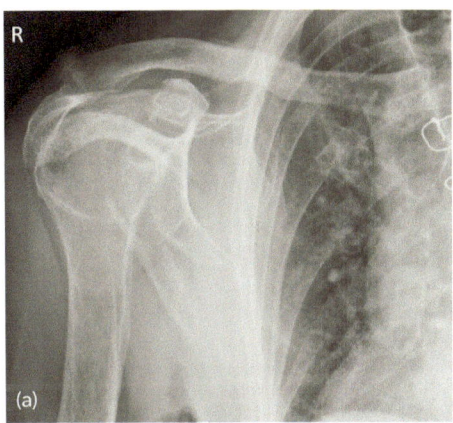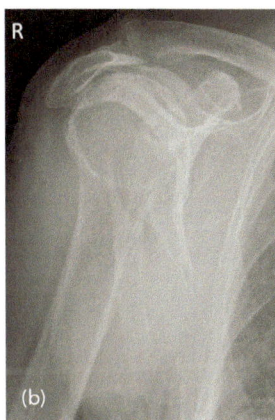

Figure 18.7 (a) Anteroposterior and (b) lateral shoulder images obtained on an 87-year-old gentleman following a fall onto the outstretched hand. The patient has dementia and there is extensive bruising on the back.

Notes:

_____

_____

_____

_____

_____

Table 18.7 Experienced reporting practitioner's detailed evaluation.

Thought process following the ABCs systematic method of evaluation	
Adequacy	The images are not technically correct; however, the patient is clearly an older patient and an abnormality is visible.
Bones	The bones are osteopenic with reduced bone density and thinned cortices. The proximal humerus, clavicle and visible ribs are intact. There is a fracture through the body of the scapula that is displaced posteriorly. This injury is normally caused by direct impact. Given the mechanism of injury is stated as a fall onto the outstretched hand, this injury is not consistent with the presented mechanism. There is extensive bruising to the back, which makes this injury suspicious.
Cartilaginous areas	The fracture line does not appear to extend to the glenoid, indicating that this is an extra-articular fracture. The head of the humerus is articulating with the glenoid cavity, indicating that there is no subluxation or dislocation. The acromioclavicular joint is normally aligned, although it does demonstrate some age-related degeneration.
Soft tissues	Only a small amount of lung field is visible, and this appears to be free from any obvious lesions. There is slight prominence to the bronchovascular markings. The patient has had heart surgery, as there are sternal wires present, so this appearance in the lungs is most likely due to heart failure.

Developing the comment		
A	Abnormality type	Fracture
B	Bone details	Scapula body
C	Cartilage involvement	Glenohumeral joint is normal; acromioclavicular joint is degenerative
D	Displacement	Posterior displacement
E	Extra features	Suspicious injury not consistent with the given mechanism. Osteopenia

Writing the comment
There is a posteriorly displaced scapula fracture; clinical correlation is needed, as injury is not consistent with history given.

PRACTICE CASE 8

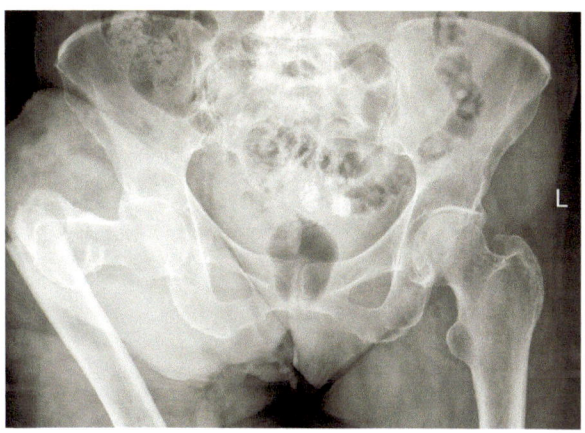

Figure 18.8 Anteroposterior pelvis image obtained following a fall downstairs. A lateral image was not obtained, as the patient was unable to elevate the left leg.

Notes:

_____

_____

_____

_____

_____

Table 18.8 Experienced reporting practitioner's detailed evaluation.

Thought process following the ABCs systematic method of evaluation	
Adequacy	A single anteroposterior pelvis has been obtained. While this is not ideal, occasionally it is not possible to acquire the standard projections and a comment needs to be made on the images obtained.
Bones	There is a fracture through the proximal femur that is angulated medially. Anteroposterior angulation or displacement cannot be assessed without a lateral image. The greater and lesser trochanters can be seen above the fracture site, making this a subtrochanteric fracture. Fractures distal to the trochanters can be pathological, so any aggressive features around the fracture need to be identified. There is no evidence of a lucent or sclerotic lesion on either side of the fracture, and the fracture margins are clearly defined and not irregular, as they might be expected should this be a pathological fracture. While a bone lesion is not visible on this image, there is superimposition of the bones and it is likely that the patient will return for further imaging of the whole femur.
Cartilaginous areas	The fracture does not involve the joint. There is some age-related degeneration in the right femoroacetabular joint. Visualised intervertebral disc spaces of the lumbar spine demonstrate degeneration.
Soft tissues	Calcifications are seen in the pelvic cavity and these are likely to be fibroids.

Developing the comment		
A	Abnormality type	Fracture
B	Bone details	Subtrochanteric region of the right femur
C	Cartilage involvement	Right hip age-related degeneration
D	Displacement	Medial angulation
E	Extra features	Fibroids

Writing the comment
There is a medially angulated subtrochanteric fracture of the right femur.

PRACTICE CASE 9

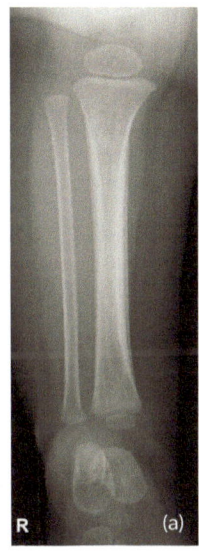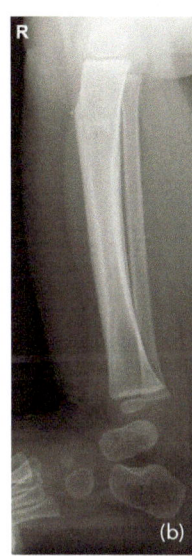

Figure 18.9 (a) Anteroposterior and (b) lateral tibia and fibula images obtained on a 2-year-old child following a fall from a slide the previous day.

Notes:

_____

_____

_____

_____

_____

Table 18.9 Experienced reporting practitioner's detailed evaluation.

Thought process following the ABCs systematic method of evaluation	
Adequacy	The images provided are adequate.
Bones	While there is no fracture visible, there is a periosteal reaction along the tibial shaft, seen on both images. The child is too old for this to be a physiological subperiosteal new bone formation, as the upper age for this is 6 months. It may be a periosteal reaction associated with a recent known injury, but the clinical history given is trauma the previous day. Thinking about the stages of fracture healing, a periosteal reaction in a young child can occur between 5 days and 3 weeks, indicating that this is not a result of injury the previous day. Alternatively, an infection or bone lesion can cause a periosteal reaction, but neither are visible on these images. This raises suspicion of neglect or an act of omission, following an injury which occurred some days earlier, such as a twisting injury leading to an undisplaced and radiologically occult spiral, or toddler's, fracture.
Cartilaginous areas	The growth plates and articular surfaces are not involved.
Soft tissues	There is some soft tissue swelling anterior to the midshaft of the tibia, seen on the lateral image, which would correlate with an injury at this site.

Developing the comment		
A	Abnormality type	Periosteal reaction but no fracture visible
B	Bone details	Midshaft of the tibia
C	Cartilage involvement	None
D	Displacement	None
E	Extra features	Appearances are not consistent with the injury provided

Writing the comment
Periosteal reaction to the midshaft of the tibia; correlation with timing of injury is needed.

PRACTICE CASE 10

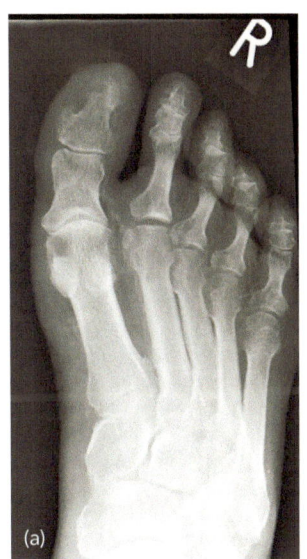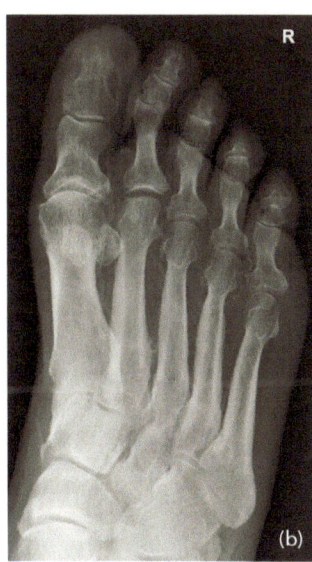

Figure 18.10 (a) Dorsi-plantar and (b) dorsi-plantar oblique toes obtained on a 67-year-old patient with diabetes with an ulcer at the tip of the big toe.

Notes:

_____

_____

_____

_____

_____

Table 18.10 Experienced reporting practitioner's detailed evaluation.

Thought process following the ABCs systematic method of evaluation	
Adequacy	The images provided are adequate.
Bones	There is some bone loss to the distal phalanx of the big toe indicating infection. Remaining bones are normal.
Cartilaginous areas	There is loss of joint space at the first metatarsophalangeal joint and the talonavicular joint, indicating age-related degeneration. It is difficult to see the second to fifth interphalangeal joints, but the remaining joint spaces are reasonably well preserved.
Soft tissues	There is no visible gas within the soft tissues, but there is some soft tissue loss at the big toe, likely where the ulcer is located. This is adjacent to the loss of bone in the distal phalanx. Vascular calcification is visible, indicating peripheral vascular disease, often seen in patients with diabetes.

Developing the comment		
A	Abnormality type	Infection
B	Bone details	First distal phalanx
C	Cartilage involvement	Age-related degeneration of the first metatarsophalangeal joint and talonavicular joint
D	Displacement	None
E	Extra features	Soft tissue changes associated with the ulcer and vascular calcification

Writing the comment
Loss of cortex and some underlying bone at the first distal phalanx in keeping with osteomyelitis; urgent onward referral.

INDEX

Note: page numbers in *italics* refer to figures, and those in **bold** to tables.